ELEVE

POCKET BOOK OF
PEDIATRIC
ANTIMICROBIAL
THERAPY

JOHN D. NELSON, M.D.

PROFESSOR OF PEDIATRICS
THE UNIVERSITY OF TEXAS
SOUTHWESTERN MEDICAL CENTER AT DALLAS
SOUTHWESTERN MEDICAL SCHOOL
DALLAS, TEXAS

Williams & Wilkins

BALTIMORE • PHILADELPHIA • HONG KONG
LONDON • MUNICH • SYDNEY • TOKYO

A WAVERLY COMPANY

Editor: Jonathan W. Pine, Jr.
Copy Editor: Stephen Seigforth
Project Manager: Barbara J. Felton

Accurate indications, adverse reactions, and dosage schedules for drugs are provided in this book, but it is possible that they may change. The reader is urged to review the package information data of the manufacturers of the medications mentioned.

Printed in the United States of America

Library of Congress Cataloging-In-Publication Data

Nelson, John D., 1930- .
  1995 Pocketbook of pediatric antimicrobial therapy/John D. Nelson.— 11th ed.
    p. cm.
  Rev. ed. of: Pocketbook of pediatric antimicrobial therapy. [1975]
  includes index.
    1. Communicable diseases in children—Chemotherapy—Handbooks, manuals, etc. 2. Antibiotics—Handbooks, manuals, etc. I. Nelson, John D., 1930- . Pocketbook of pediatric antimicrobial therapy. II. Title.
    [DNLM: 1. Antibiotics—therapeutic use—handbooks. 2. Drug Therapy—in infancy & childhood—handbooks. QV 39 N427p]
  RJ53.A5N44 1989 615.5'8—dc19 88-26186
    ISBN 0-683-06406-1

                                              95 96 97 98
                                           3 4 5 6 7 8 9 10

TABLE OF CONTENTS

I. INTRODUCTION TO THE ELEVENTH EDITION

This book is revised every two years. The field of infectious disease is constantly growing and changing. New diseases are discovered, new antimicrobials are introduced, older antibiotics lose their utility for certain diseases but sometimes find new applications and microbes find ways to escape the action of antimicrobials. Each time I revise this book I wonder at the extent of changes that are necessary.

I appreciate greatly the helpful criticisms and suggestions of my infectious disease colleagues at The University of Texas Southwestern Medical Center: George McCracken, Trudy Murphy, Mahmoud Mustafa, Octavio Ramilo, Pablo Sanchez and Jane Siegel. I extend special thanks to John Bennett for reviewing the antifungal section and to Pablo Sanchez for help with the newborn section.

Recent editions of this book have been translated into Chinese, Indonesian, Italian, Polish, Portuguese and Spanish. This task of the translators is complicated by the variability of drug availability in different countries. Fortunately, the major antimicrobials are universally available.

The large numbers of related drugs mean that multiple options are available for a great many diseases. To avoid cluttering up and expanding the book I have indicated only one or two options for treating most infections. Clearly, other regimens might be suitable.

Some dosages and indications differ from those in the manufacturers' package inserts. In such situations the dosages recommended in this book have been found by controlled studies or by clinical experience to be efficacious and safe.

The continued popularity and apparent utility of this little book is gratifying. As in the past, I encourage you to send suggestions for its improvement to me.

John D. Nelson, M.D.

II. CHOOSING AMONG AMINOGLYCOSIDES, BETA-LACTAMS AND MACROLIDES

New drugs should be compared with others in the same class regarding (1) antimicrobial spectrum, (2) degree of potency within the spectrum, (3) pharmacokinetic properties, (4) demonstrated efficacy in clinical trials, (5) tolerance, toxicity and side effects, and (6) cost. If there is no substantial benefit in any of those areas, one should opt for staying with the older, more familiar drug because of the risk of unexpected adverse effects inherent in any new product.

Aminoglycosides. Five aminoglycosidic antibiotics are available in the U.S. as major drugs for coliform bacillary infections: amikacin, gentamicin, kanamycin, netilmicin and tobramycin. (Streptomycin and spectinomycin have limited uses.) Resistance of Gram-negative bacilli to aminoglycosides is caused by adenylating, acetylating or phosphorylating enzymes produced by the bacteria which inactivate the antibiotic. The specific activities are highly variable. As a result, antibiotic susceptibility tests must be done for each aminoglycoside drug separately. Kanamycin is not effective against *Pseudomonas aeruginosa* so the others are preferred whenever that infection is present or suspected. There are small differences in comparative toxicities of these aminoglycosides to the kidneys and eighth cranial nerve. In animal models netilmicin is the least toxic. It is possible that netilmicin and tobramycin are the safest, but there are conflicting reports in studies focusing on small changes in renal function rather than on frank renal failure. It is uncertain whether or not these small differences are clinically significant. In any case, it is advisable to monitor peak and trough serum concentrations in all patients; elevated peak and trough concentrations correlate with toxicity. Desired peak concentrations with amikacin and kanamycin are 20-35 μg/ml and trough concentrations less than 10 μg/ml; for the others they are 5-10 μg/ml and less than 2 μg/ml, respectively. Patients with cystic fibrosis require larger than normal dosage to achieve therapeutic serum concentrations and they excrete aminoglycosides more rapidly. In the case of nosocomial infection, the choice among aminoglycosides should be based on knowledge of local susceptibility patterns. In addition to routine monitoring of *in vitro* susceptibility testing results to detect emergence of resistant strains, the policy of switching among the drugs for routine hospital use every one to two years might minimize the likelihood of resistance due to selective drug pressure.

Oral Cephalosporins (Cefaclor, cefadroxil, cefixime, cefpodoxime, cefprozil, ceftibuten, cefuroxime axetil, cephalexin, cephradine and loracarbef). As a class, the oral cephalosporins have the advantages over oral penicillins of somewhat greater safety and greater palatability of the suspension formulations. (Penicillins have a bitter taste.) Cefuroxime and cefpodoxime are the least palatable. Cephalexin and cephradine have virtually identical properties and effectiveness and can be used interchangeably. The half-lives of cefadroxil, cefpodoxime, cefprozil, ceftibuten and loracarbef in serum are about twice as long as those of the other drugs. This pharmacokinetic feature accounts for the fact that they can be given in only one or two daily doses. Cefaclor, cefixime, cefpodoxime, cefprozil, ceftibuten, loracarbef and cefuroxime have the advantage of adding *Haemophilus influenzae* (including beta-lactamase-producing strains) to the spectrum. The newer oral cephalosporins have decreased activity against staphylococci.

Parenteral Cephalosporins. First generation cephalosporins (cefazolin, cephalothin, cephapirin, cephradine) have limited application in pediatrics. They have been used mainly as back-up drugs for treatment of Gram-positive infections because their Gram-negative spectrum is limited. Cefazolin is tolerated best on intramuscular injection; furthermore, it is given q8h because of its longer half-life in serum rather than on the q4-6h schedules used for the others. Differences in the frequencies of vein irritation among the group are minor.

The second generation cephalosporins (cefamandole and cefuroxime) and the cephamycin (cefoxitin) added to the antibacterial spectrum. Cefoxitin has good activity against *Bacteroides fragilis* and can be used in place of chloramphenicol or clindamycin when that organism is implicated in disease. Cefotetan has a spectrum similar to that of cefoxitin but a longer serum half-life, so it can be given q12h. Cefamandole and cefuroxime added *Haemophilus influenzae* to the spectrum of cephalosporins. However, cefamandole is somewhat unstable to the TEM1 beta-lactamase elaborated by *H. influenzae*. This combined with its rather poor penetration into cerebrospinal fluid resulted in cases of *Haemophilus* meningitis developing in infants being treated with cefamandole. Cefuroxime is more stable to the enzyme and has better penetration into CSF (comparable to that of ampicillin). It has been used to treat meningitis due to the usual pathogens; however, reports of delayed sterilization of CSF limit its use for meningitis. Cefuroxime has utility as single drug therapy (in place of combinations such as nafcillin and chloramphenicol) for infants and young children with pneumonia, bone and joint infections or other conditions in which Gram-positive cocci and *Haemophilus* are the usual pathogens. Cefonicid has a prolonged serum half-life so that doses can be given every 12-24 hours. Cefonicid is not approved for use in children.

Among the many so-called third generation cephalosporins, cefoperazone is not yet approved for use in children. All have enhanced potency against many Gram-negative bacilli, usually including aminoglycoside resistant organisms. They are inactive against enterococci and *Listeria* and have variable activity against *Pseudomonas* and *Bacteroides*. Cefotaxime and ceftriaxone have been used successfully to treat meningitis caused by the usual pathogens. Limited experience with ceftazidime and ceftizoxime suggests they too are effective for meningitis. These drugs have greatest utility for treating Gram-negative bacillary infections when aminoglycosides are contraindicated or when the organisms are resistant to customarily used drugs. Because cefoperazone and ceftriaxone are excreted to a large extent via the liver, they can be used with little dosage adjustment in patients with renal failure. Ceftazidime has the unique property of activity against *Pseudomonas aeruginosa* that is comparable to that of the aminoglycosides. Ceftriaxone has a serum half-life of 4-7 hours and can be given once or twice a day.

Penicillinase-resistant Penicillins (Cloxacillin, dicloxacillin, methicillin, nafcillin, oxacillin). Nafcillin differs pharmacologically from the others in being excreted primarily by the liver rather than by the kidneys. This may be the reason for its lack of nephrotoxicity. Nephrotoxicity or hemorrhagic cystitis occurs in 5% of children treated with methicillin. For this reason nafcillin is preferred over methicillin or oxacillin for parenteral use with two exceptions: the neonate and patients with hepatic disease. Nafcillin pharmacokinetics in the newborn are erratic, especially in jaundiced babies; furthermore, methicillin nephrotoxicity is rare in the neonate. Nafcillin pharmacokinetics are also erratic in persons with liver disease. For oral use, cloxacillin, oxacillin and dicloxacillin are essentially equivalent, but the latter has the greatest anti-staphylococcal activity *in vitro*.

Anti-pseudomonal Penicillins (Azlocillin, imipenem, mezlocillin, piperacillin, ticarcillin, ticarcillin-clavulanate). Azlocillin and piperacillin are the most active *in vitro* against *Pseudomonas*. (Azlocillin is not available in the U.S.) Mezlocillin does not affect platelet adhesiveness significantly, but the others do; this could be an advantage in patients who have another risk factor for bleeding. In general, *Pseudomonas* strains resistant to ticarcillin are resistant to the newer drugs. These drugs should be used along with an aminoglycoside or cephalosporin for treating *Pseudomonas* infections in compromised hosts for synergistic effect. Timentin® is the combination of ticarcillin and the beta-lactamase inhibitor, clavulanate and Zosyn® is the combination of piperacillin with tazobactam, another beta-lactamase inhibitor. The combinations have little effect on activity against *Pseudomonas* but do extend the spectrum to many beta-lactamase-positive bacteria. Imipenem is a carbapenem with a broader spectrum of activity than any other beta-lactam currently available. It is not approved by the FDA for use in children and experience with it is limited. At present it is recommended for treatment of infections caused by bacteria resistant to all other drugs.

Aminopenicillins (Amoxicillin, amoxicillin-clavulanate, ampicillin, ampicillin-sulbactam, bacampicillin, cyclacillin). Bacampicillin is rapidly and completely converted in the body to ampicillin so it is an indirect means of administering ampicillin. Bacampicillin and cyclacillin are the most efficiently absorbed so peak blood concentrations are greater than after the same dosage of amoxicillin or ampicillin. Ampicillin is more likely than the others to cause diarrhea and to disturb colonic coliform flora and cause overgrowth of *Candida*. Augmentin® is a combination of amoxicillin and clavulanate for oral use that permits amoxicillin to be active against many beta-lactamase-producing bacteria. Sulbactam, another beta-lactamase inhibitor, is combined with ampicillin in the parenteral formulation, Unasyn®. Clinical experience is too limited to date to assess its role in pediatric patients.

Monobactams. The only monobactam licensed for use in the U.S. is aztreonam. Its spectrum is similar to that of the anti-*Pseudomonas* aminoglycosides so the clinical indications are similar. Experience with the drug to date is insufficient to know for which clinical situations, if any, that it might replace the aminoglycosides.

4

Macrolides. Erythromycin is the prototype of a class called macrolide antibiotics. Almost thirty macrolides have been produced, but only three are commercially available in the U.S.: erythromycin, azithromycin and clarithromycin. (Azithromycin is actually an azalide compound structurally similar to macrolides.) As a class these drugs achieve greater concentrations in tissues than in serum. (Tissue concentrations are markedly greater with azithromycin and clarithromycin than with erythromycin.) As a result, measuring serum concentrations is clinically not useful. Erythromycin has poor gastrointestinal tolerance in many patients. This is less of a problem with the newer drugs. Erythromycin suspensions are ester formulations and must be hydrolyzed to the active base compound. The estolate form results in greater serum and tissue concentrations of erythromycin than do the other esters. Macrolides have the broadest range of antimicrobial activity of all classes of antibiotics. This is especially true of azithromycin and clarithromycin which are demonstrating clinical utility in *Haemophilus influenzae,* chlamydial and mycobacterial infections greater than that of erythromycin.

III. PENICILLIN DESENSITIZATION

Studies have shown that an oral regimen is safer and more effective than graduated injections for desensitization to penicillins. (**Pediatr Infect Dis** 1982;1:344)

Penicillin V suspension is used. Signed, informed consent is recommended. An intravenous line is in place and emergency resuscitation materials at hand for the unlikely event of anaphylaxis. A physician should be in attendance. Doses are given at 15 minute intervals; the total regimen requires 4 hours.

Doses	Penicillin V units/ml	Amount q15 min
1-7	1,000	Doubling doses from 0.1 ml (100 units) to 6.4 ml (6,400 units)
8-10	10,000	Doubling doses from 1.2 ml (12,000 units) to 4.8 ml (48,000 units)
11-14	80,000	Doubling doses from 1.0 ml (80,000 units) to 8.0 ml (640,000 units)

(Reference: **N Engl J Med** 1985;312:1229)

Minor allergic reactions are suppressed with epinephrine or antihistamines. Therapy is not interrupted unless there is a severe or unsuppressible reaction. If there are interruptions in therapy of more than 8 hours, it is advisable to repeat the desensitization regimen.

If the patient cannot tolerate oral medication, parenteral desensitization can be used. The method is reviewed in **J Allergy Clin Immunol** 1982;69:275.

IV. SEQUENTIAL PARENTERAL-ORAL ANTIBIOTIC THERAPY FOR SERIOUS INFECTIONS

Bacterial pneumonias, endocarditis and bone and joint infections often require prolonged antibiotic therapy. Intravenous therapy not only is unpleasant for the child but carries a hazard of serious nosocomial disease.

Rationale:
1. Comparable dosages of analogous parenteral and oral medications result in comparable serum concentrations from 1 to 6 hours after a dose and comparable bioavailability ("area-under-the-curve") in most patients.
2. There is no known therapeutic advantage to the momentary high serum concentrations during IV administration.
3. Although the protein binding of many oral formulations is greater than that of parenteral formulations, this does not prevent good penetration into body fluid compartments.

Method:
1. Initial parenteral therapy
   a. Alert laboratory to save pathogen for serum bactericidal tests.
   b. Perform any necessary surgical procedures.
2. Subsequent oral therapy when clinical condition is stable and patient is able to take and retain oral medication
   a. Select appropriate oral antibiotic based on *in vitro* susceptibilities and compliance factors (mainly palatability of suspension formulations).
   b. BEGIN WITH DOSAGE 2-3 TIMES "NORMAL" DOSAGE: e.g. 75-100 MG/KG/DAY OF DICLOXACILLIN AND 100-150 MG/KG/DAY OF OTHER BETA-LACTAMS.
   c. Serum for bactericidal titer or measurement of antibiotic concentration 1-2 hours after a dose.

NOTES:
1. The serum bactericidal titer is done quantitatively and is defined as ≥ 99.9% killing (100% killing is seldom achieved). For staphylococcal or *Haemophilus* infections the serum bactericidal titer should be at least 1:8. For highly susceptible bacteria such as pneumococci and Group A streptococci, titers are usually greater than 1:32. Peak serum antibiotic concentration should be ≥ 20 μg/ml for beta-lactams and ≥ 10 μg/ml for clindamycin.
2. Peak serum activity usually is found 45-60 minutes after a dose taken as suspension and 1-2 hours after a capsule or tablet.
3. Approximately 5-10% of patients are unsuitable for this regimen because of poor GI absorption of antibiotics.

WARNING: ORAL THERAPY REGIMENS FOR SERIOUS INFECTIONS ARE POTENTIALLY HAZARDOUS UNLESS ADEQUACY OF SERUM BACTERICIDAL ACTIVITY IS MONITORED.

V. ANTIBIOTIC THERAPY FOR NEWBORNS

A. RECOMMENDED THERAPY FOR SELECTED CONDITIONS

NOTE: To avoid repetition, the recommended dosages and intervals of administration of antibiotics indicated with an asterisk in most of the following conditions are given in the Table on pages 16 and 17.

Condition	Therapy	Comment
Congenital syphilis	Penicillin G 50,000 u/kg q 12h (day of life 1-7), q8h (>7 days) IV OR procaine penicillin G 50,000 u/kg/day IM daily x 10-14 days	Obtain follow-up serology at 3,6,12 mos until nontreponemal test nonreactive
Congenital toxoplasmosis	Trisulfapyrimidines or sulfadiazine 100 mg/kg/day PO div q12h AND pyrimethamine 1 mg/kg PO once daily for 3 days, then every other day; x 12 mos	Supplemental folinic acid 5-10 mg every 3 days during pyrimethamine administration
Herpes simplex infection	Acyclovir 30 mg/kg/day as 1-2 hr IV infusion div q8h OR vidarabine 15-30 mg/kg/day as 12 hour or longer IV infusion x 10 days; PLUS trifluoridine ophthalmic sol'n topically q2h for conjunctivitis	Larger dosages of acyclovir and longer duration of Rx are being tested
Tetanus neonatorum	Penicillin G* IV x 10 days	Antitoxin and sedation; Do not use IM injections
Parotitis, suppurative	Methicillin* IV AND aminoglycoside IV, IM x 10 days	Usually staphylococcal but occasionally coliform

8

- Gonococcal	Ceftriaxone 50 mg/kg/day (max. 125 mg) IV, IM once daily OR cefotaxime 50 mg/kg/day IV, IM div q12h; x 7 days (A single dose of ceftriaxone may be effective in uncomplicated infection)	days OR topical erythromycin, tetracycline or sulfacetamide ointment q.i.d. topical therapy because NP carrier state eradicated; Treat mother and her sexual partner with tetracycline Chloramphenicol or tetra-cycline ophthalmic drops or ointment optional but not necessary; Treat mother and her sexual partner
- Staphylococcus aureus	Methicillin* IM, IV x 7-10 days	Additionally: Neomycin ophthalmic drops or ointment (systemic antibiotic not used for minor infection)
- Pseudomonas aeruginosa	Ticarcillin* or mezlocillin* IV, IM AND amino-glycoside* IM, IV x 7-10 days (Alternative: ceftazidime*)	Polymyxin B ophthalmic drops or ointment; Subtenon or subconjunctival antibiotics in some cases
Gastrointestinal Infections		
- Enteropathogenic E. coli	Neomycin 100 mg/kg/day PO div q8h x 5 days	Most "enteropathogenic" strains neither toxigenic nor invasive
- Salmonella	Cefotaxime* IV, IM x 7-10 days if suspected sepsis or focal infection	Observe for focal complications (meningitis, arthritis, etc.)

* See pages 16-17 for dosage

NEWBORN

9

NEWBORN

Condition	Therapy	Comment
- Necrotizing enterocolitis or peritonitis secondary to bowel rupture	Ticarcillin* IV, IM AND aminoglycoside* IM, IV x 10 days or longer; cefotaxime* suitable alternative to aminoglycoside; vancomycin* IV if *S. epidermidis* or methicillin-resistant staphylococcus cultured; common alternative: vancomycin* + clindamycin*	Bacteremia in 30-50% of cases; After 2-3 days of age *Bacteroides* common in gut; Clindamycin* or metronidazole* for ticarcillin-resistant *B. fragilis*
Sepsis and Meningitis	NOTE: Dexamethasone adjunctive therapy for meningitis is currently being evaluated in neonates	Duration of therapy: 7-10 days for sepsis without a focus; 21 days minimum for meningitis
- Initial therapy, organism unknown	Ampicillin* IV AND aminoglycoside* IV, IM	Ampicillin* AND cefotaxime* is a suitable alternative, especially if aminoglycoside-resistant nosocomial organism suspected
- *Bacteroides fragilis* spp. *fragilis*	Metronidazole*, clindamycin*, mezlocillin* or ticarcillin* IV, IM	Metronidazole preferred for CNS infection
- Coliform bacteria	Cefotaxime* IV, IM; Lumbar intrathecal or intraventricular injections of aminoglycoside are not beneficial in usual case	Aminoglycoside* is suitable alternative
- Group A or nonerterococcal Group D streptccocci	Penicillin G* IV	
- Group B streptococcus	Ampicillin* or penicillin G* IV AND gentamicin* IV IM (Discontinue gentamicin when strain known to be fully susceptible to ampicillin)	Synergy may be advantage esp against penicillin-tolerant strains

10

Organism	Treatment	Notes
- *Staphylococcus epidermidis*	Vancomycin* IV	Many methicillin-resistant
- *Staphylococcus aureus*	Methicillin* IV, IM; Vancomycin* IV for methicillin-resistant *Staphylococcus*	Rarely causes meningitis in newborn; Vancomycin preferred for meningitis
- *Pseudomonas aeruginosa*	Mezlocillin* or ticarcillin* IV, IM AND aminoglycoside* IV, IM	Ceftazidime* is a suitable alternative

Osteomyelitis, Suppurative Arthritis

Organism	Treatment	Notes
- Gonococcal arthritis and tenosynovitis	Ceftriaxone* IV, IM x 7-10 days (penicillin G* IV if organism susceptible)	Surgical drainage of pus; early institution of physical therapy
- *Staphylococcus aureus*	Methicillin* IV, IM x 21 days minimum; Vancomycin* IV for methicillin-resistant *Staphylococcus*	Change to penicillin G if organism susceptible
- Coliform bacteria	Cefotaxime* OR aminoglycoside* IV, IM x 21 days minimum	Cephalosporins better than aminoglycosides for deep tissue infection
- Group B streptococcus	(See Group B streptococcal meningitis)	
- Unknown	Methicillin* IV, IM AND cefotaxime* IV, IM x 21 days minimum	

11

* See pages 16-17 for dosage

NEWBORN

Condition	Therapy	Comment
Otitis Media	Few controlled treatment trials in newborns; Suggest using initial therapy as for older infants (see page 24); If no response, obtain middle ear fluid for culture	Cefaclor or Augmentin may have advantage because of activity vs. coliforms and Staph which cause disease in 10-20% of cases
- Coliform bacteria	Cefaclor 30-40 mg/kg/day PO div q8-12h x 10 days OR Augmentin (same dosage)	Aminoglycoside* or cefotaxime* if parenteral therapy needed
- *Staphylococcus aureus*	Cloxacillin 50 mg/kg/day PO div q6-8h x 10 days	Methicillin* if unable to treat PO
- Streptococcus (incl. pneumococcus)	Penicillin V 30 mg/kg/day PO div q8h x 10 days	Given IV, IM for complicated otitis
- *Haemophilus*	Cefaclor 30-40 mg/kg/day PO div q8-12h OR amoxicillin 30-40 mg/kg/day PO div q8-12h if susceptible	Other regimens not tested in neonates
Pulmonary Infections		
- *Staphylococcus aureus*	Methicillin* IV, IM x 21 days minimum; Vancomycin* IV for methicillin-resistant Staph	Closed tube drainage of empyema
- *Pseudomonas aeruginosa*	Mezlocillin* or ticarcillin* IV, IM AND aminoglycoside* IV, IM x 14 days or longer	Ceftazidime* is a suitable alternative
- Group B streptococcus	Penicillin G* IV OR ampicillin* IV, IM x 10-14 days	Radiograph often mimics hyaline membrane disease
- *Chlamydia trachomatis*	Erythromycin* PO x 14-21 days	Ampicillin, amoxicillin or sulfa drugs may be effective

Condition	Treatment	Comments
		pneumonia and do not require antibiotic therapy
- Pertussis	Erythromycin* x 5-10 days OR ampicillin* IV, IM if PO meds not retained	Usually acquired from parent or other adult in household
Skin and Soft Tissues		
- Impetigo neonatorum	Cleansing alone OR methicillin* IV, IM OR cephalexin 50 mg/kg/day PO div q6-8h OR mupirocin topically; x 5 days	No antibiotic for superficial impetigo; Chlorhexidine baths; Break lesions with alcohol swab
- Erysipelas (and other Group A streptococcal infections)	Penicillin G* IV x 5-7 days	Group B streptococcus may produce similar cellulitis or nodular lesions
- Breast abscess	Methicillin* IV, IM x 5-7 days; aminoglycoside* OR cefotaxime* if Gram-negative rods seen in pus	Gram stain of expressed pus/colostrum or I&D material necessary to select initial therapy; I&D of pus (Avoid damage to breast tissue)
- Staphylococcus	Methicillin* IV, IM x 5-7 days; vancomycin* for methicillin-resistant Staphylococcus	Value of systemic antibiotics over surgical drainage alone not established
- Group B streptococcus	Penicillin G* IV OR ampicillin* IV, IM x 5-7 days	Usually no pus formed
- Coliform bacteria	Aminoglycoside* IM, IV x 5-7 days; Alternative: cefotaxime*	

* See pages 16-17 for dosage

NEWBORN

13

NEWBORN

Condition	Therapy	Comment
Skin and Soft Tissues (cont.)		
- Omphalitis and funisitis		
Group A or B streptococci	Penicillin G* IV x 5-7 days OR (for Group A strep) benzathine penicillin G 50,000 u/kg IM x 1 dose PLUS topical "triple dye" or bacitracin ointment	Group A strep usually causes "wet cord" without pus and with minimal erythema
Staphylococcus aureus	Methicillin* IV, IM x 5 days or longer	Observe for bacteremia and other focus of infection
Necrotizing funisitis	Methicillin* IV, IM AND aminoglycoside* IV, IM	Unknown etiology but coliform or staphylococcal secondary infection may occur
Clostridial	Penicillin G* IV x 10 days or longer	Crepitance and rapidly spreading cellulitis around umbilicus
Urinary Tract Infection		LARGER DOSAGES OF DRUGS REQUIRED IF ACCOMPANYING SEPSIS: Investigate for anomalies of urinary tract
- Coliform bacteria	Gentamicin 3 mg/kg/day IV, IM div q12h OR amikacin 10 mg/kg/day IV, IM div q12h x 10 days	Ampicillin used for *Proteus mirabilis* infection
- *Pseudomonas aeruginosa*	Mezlocillin or ticarcillin IV, IM 75-100 mg/kg/day IV, IM div q8-12h	Ceftazidime* is a suitable alternative
- Enterococcus	Ampicillin 30 mg/kg/day IV, IM or 50 mg/kg/day PO div q8h x 10 days	If culture remains positive, add an aminoglycoside for synergistic effect

14

A number of factors determine the degree of transfer of antibiotics across the placenta: lipid solubility, degree of ionization, molecular weight, protein binding, placental maturation, and placental and fetal blood flow. During the latter part of pregnancy maternal serum concentrations of most antibiotics decrease because of the increased volume of distribution. Fetal serum concentrations of the following drugs are equal to, or only slightly less than, those in the mother: penicillin G, amoxicillin, ampicillin, carbenicillin, methicillin, sulfonamides, trimethoprim, tetracyclines, nitrofurantoin and chloramphenicol. The aminoglycoside concentrations in fetal serum are from 20-50% of those in maternal serum. Cephalosporins, nafcillin, oxacillin, clindamycin and colistimethate penetrate poorly (10-15%) and fetal concentrations of erythromycin and dicloxacillin are less than 10% of those in the mother.

Some drugs can cause harm to the pregnant woman or fetus. Drugs that are <u>contraindicated</u> are: ribavirin, amantadine, cinoxacin, ciprofloxacin, norfloxacin, erythromycin estolate, griseofulvin, nalidixic acid, tetracyclines, emetine, lindane and primaquine. Drugs that are <u>considered safe</u> are: penicillins, aztreonam, cephalosporins, erythromycin base, methenamine mandelate, spectinomycin, nystatin, chloroquine, niclosamide, paromomycin, permethrin, praziquantel, pyrantel pamoate and pyrethrins. Drugs not listed should be used with caution for firm clinical indications. (**The Medical Letter** 1987;29:61).

Concentrations of antibiotics in human breast milk are not well studied. Isoniazid, metronidazole, trimethoprim and sulfonamides occur in equal concentrations in maternal serum and milk. Tetracyclines, chloramphenicol and erythromycin are found in breast milk in concentrations 50-75% of those in serum. Breast milk concentrations of penicillin G and V, aminoglycosides, nalidixic acid, oxacillin, novobiocin, various cephalosporins, and nitrofurantoin have been reported to be less than 25% of the maternal serum concentrations. Because these are microgram amounts they would not be ingested by the infant in therapeutic amounts.

For example, if an infant took 110 cc/kg body weight of breast milk containing 10 mcg/ml isoniazid in a day, this would amount to a "dose" of 1.1 mg/kg/day. The same infant ingesting milk containing 10 mg/dl of sulfonamide would receive 11 mg/kg/day. On the other hand, with a penicillin V concentration of 0.1 mcg/ml in breast milk, the amount of penicillin taken in by the infant would be only 0.011 mg/kg/day.

The AAP Committee on Drugs recommends that breast feeding be discontinued 12-24 hours before treating a nursing mother with metronidazole. Other antibiotics are usually compatible with breast feeding but it warns about the possibility of inducing hemolysis in babies with G-6-PD deficiency by nalidixic acid, nitrofurantoin or sulfa drugs. (Transfer of Drugs and Other Chemicals into Human Milk. **Pediatrics** 1994;93:137)

NEWBORN

C. TABLE OF ANTIBIOTIC DOSAGES FOR NEONATES

Antibiotics	Routes	Weight <1200 g Age 0-4 wk	Weight 1200-2000 g Age 0-7 days	>7 days	Weight > 2000 g Age 0-7 days	>7 days
Amikacin	IV, IM	7.5 q18-24h	7.5 q12-18h	7.5 q8-12h	10 q12h	10 q8h
Ampicillin	IV, IM					
Meningitis		50 q12h	50 q12h	50 q8h	50 q8h	50 q6h
Other diseases		25 q12h	25 q12h	25 q8h	25 q8h	25 q6h
Aztreonam	IV, IM	30 q12h	30 q12h	30 q8h	30 q8h	30 q6h
Cefazolin	IV, IM	20 q12h	20 q12h	20 q12h	20 q12h	20 q8h
Cefotaxime	IV, IM	50 q12h	50 q12h	50 q8h	50 q12h	50 q8h
Ceftazidime	IV, IM	50 q12h	50 q12h	50 q8h	50 q8h	50 q8h
Ceftriaxone	IV, IM	50 q24h	50 q24h	50 q24h	50 q24h	75 q24h
Cephalothin	IV	20 q12h	20 q12h	20 q8h	20 q8h	20 q6h
Chloramphenicol	IV, PO	25 q24h	25 q24h	25 q24h	25 q24h	25 q12h
Clindamycin	IV, IM, PO	5 q12h	5 q12h	5 q8h	5 q8h	5 q6h
Erythromycin	PO	10 q12h	10 q12h	10 q8h	10 q12h	10 q8h
Gentamicin	IV, IM	2.5 q18-24h	2.5 q12-18h	2.5 q8-12h	2.5 q12h	2.5 q8h
Imipenem	IV, IM	20 q18-24h	20 q12h	20 q12h	20 q12h	20 q8h
	IV, IM	7.5 q18-24h	7.5 q12h	7.5 q8-12h	10 q12h	10 q8h

	Route					
Meningitis		50 q12h	50 q12h	50 q8h	50 q8h	50 q6h
Other diseases		25 q12h	25 q12h	25 q8h	25 q8h	25 q6h
Metronidazole	IV, PO	7.5 q48h	7.5 q24h	7.5 q12h	7.5 q12h	15 q12h
Mezlocillin	IV, IM	75 q12h	75 q12h	75 q8h	75 q12h	75 q8h
Oxacillin	IV, IM	25 q12h	25 q12h	25 q8h	25 q8h	25 q6h
Nafcillin	IV	25 q12h	25 q12h	25 q8h	25 q8h	25 q6h
Netilmicin	IV, IM	2.5 q18-24h	2.5 q12-18h	2.5 q8-12h	2.5 q12h	2.5 q8h
Penicillin G Meningitis	IV	50,000 u q12h	50,000 u q12h	75,000 u q8h	50,000 u q8h	50,000 u q6h
Other diseases		25,000 u q12h	25,000 u q12h	25,000 u q8h	25,000 u q8h	25,000 u q6h
Penicillin G Benzathine	IM		50,000 u (one dose)	50,000 u (one dose)	50,000 u (one dose)	50,000 u (one dose)
Procaine			50,000 u q24h	50,000 u q24h	50,000 u q24h	50,000 u q24
Ticarcillin	IV, IM	75 q12h	75 q12h	75 q8h	75 q8h	75 q6h
Tobramycin	IV, IM	2.5 q18-24h	2.5 q12-18h	2.5 q8-12h	2.5 q12h	2.5 q8h
Vancomycin	IV	15 q24h	15 q12-18h	15 q8-12h	15 q12h	15 q8h

Recommendations for infants weighing <1200 g based on Prober et al, **Pediatr Infect Dis J** 1990;9:111

VI. ANTIMICROBIAL THERAPY ACCORDING TO CLINICAL SYNDROMES

NOTES:

1. This tabulation should be considered a rough guideline for the "average" patient. Deviations should be made according to physiologic peculiarities of the patient. Dosages recommended are for patients with normal or nearly normal hydration, renal function and hepatic function. See Section XII for patients with impaired renal function and Section XV for dosages based on square meters of body surface area.

2. Duration of treatment should be individualized. The periods recommended are based on common practice and general experience. Critical evaluations of duration of therapy have been carried out in very few diseases.

3. Diseases are arranged by body systems. Consult the index for the alphabetized listing of diseases and Section VII for the alphabetized listing of etiologic agents and for uncommon agents not included in this Section.

Clinical Diagnosis	Therapy	Comments
A. SKIN AND SOFT TISSUE INFECTIONS		
Streptococcal cellulitis (erysipelas)	Penicillin G 50,000-100,000 u/kg/day, IV div q4-6h initially; then penicillin V 50 mg (80,000 u)/kg/day PO div q6-8h x 10 days	NOTE: Erythromycin for penicillin-allergic patients These dosages may be un-necessarily large but little clinical experience with smaller dosages
Lymphangitis, lympha-denitis, blistering dactylitis (streptococcal)	Penicillin V 25-50 mg (40,000-80,000 u)/kg/day PO div q6-8h OR erythromycin 40-50 mg/kg/day PO div q8-12h; x 10 days	For severe disease, penicillin IV (as above)
Impetigo	Mupirocin topically to lesions t.i.d.; OR (for extensive lesions) erythromycin (as above) or cefadroxil 30 mg/kg/day PO div q12h	Bathe daily; Usually mixed streptococcal and staphylococcal infection
Bullous impetigo, staphylococcal scarlet fever	Cefadroxil 30 mg/kg/day PO div q12h OR cloxacillin 50 mg/kg/day PO div q6h x 5-7 days	Other anti-staphylococcal drugs can be used

18

Condition	Treatment	Notes
Scalded skin syndrome	Nafcillin (or related drug) 150 mg/kg/day IV div q6h initially; then cloxacillin OR cefadroxil (as above) x 5-7 days	Burow's or Zephiran compresses for intertriginous areas
Pyoderma, abscesses, cervical adenitis, Ludwig's angina (streptococcal, staphylococcal)	Cefadroxil OR cloxacillin (as above); x5-10 days	I & D when indicated; Nafcillin IV for serious infections
Necrotizing fasciitis (streptococcal, staphylococcal)	Nafcillin 150 mg/kg/day IV div q6h x 10 days (add aminoglycoside or ceftazidime if Gram-negative infection suspected)	Debridement; Watch for hypocalcemia, hypoproteinemia; Occasionally due to Gram-negative organisms
Buccal cellulitis (*Haemophilus*) or cellulitis of unknown etiology	Cefotaxime 100-150 mg/kg/day IV div q6h OR ceftriaxone 50 mg/kg IM, IV once daily; OR chloramphenicol 50-75 mg/kg/day IV, x 5-7 days	R/O meningitis; LARGER DOSAGES NEEDED FOR MENINGITIS
Suppurative myositis (Staphylococcal) (Syn: tropical myositis, pyomyositis)	Nafcillin 150 mg/kg/day IV div q6h x 7-10 days Alternatives: other anti-staphylococcal beta-lactams, vancomycin	Surgical drainage or excision when needed
Gas gangrene (clostridial)	Penicillin G 250,000 u/kg/day IV div q4h x 10 days; Consider hyperbaric oxygen therapy	Antitoxin was of doubtful efficacy and is no longer available
Non-tuberculous (atypical) mycobacterial adenitis	Total surgical excision is usually curative and antimicrobial therapy is not necessary	If surgical excision not possible, rifampin or clarithromycin therapy possibly effective
Tuberculous adenitis	As for pulmonary tuberculosis (See page 26)	Surgical excision usually not indicated

Clinical Diagnosis	Therapy	Comments
Animal and human bites	Augmentin 20-40 mg/kg/day PO div q8h x 5-7 days	Human bites often mixed aerobes and anaerobes; Consider rabies prophylaxis for animal bites; Tetanus prophylaxis
B. SKELETAL INFECTIONS		SEE SECTION IV FOR DISCUSSION OF ORAL ANTIBIOTIC THERAPY
Suppurative arthritis		Needle aspiration or surgical open drainage; Physiotherapy
- Newborns	See Section V	
- Infants (*Haemophilus*, streptococci, *Staphylococcus*)	Cefuroxime or cefotaxime 100-150 mg/kg/day IV, IM div q8h OR (for streptococcus) penicillin G 100,000 u/kg/day IV div q4-6h x 14 days or longer OR (for *Staphylococcus*) nafcillin 150 mg/kg/day IV div q6h; x 21 days or longer	Perform LP in patients with *Haemophilus*; LARGER DOSAGES NEEDED FOR MENINGITIS
- Children (*Staphylococcus*, streptococci)	Nafcillin 150 mg/kg/day IV div q6h x 3 weeks or longer; Alternatives: other beta-lactams, clindamycin; vancomycin for methicillin-resistant staphylococci	Change to penicillin G if streptococcus or susceptible pneumococcus
- Gonococcal arthritis or tenosynovitis	Ceftriaxone 50 mg/kg once daily IV, IM OR (if susceptible) penicillin G 100,000 u/kg/day IV div q6h x 7-10 days	3-5 days therapy adequate in adults, but not tested in children
- Other bacteria	See Section VII for preferred antibiotics	

20

Osteomyelitis or osteochondritis

- Newborn | See Section V | Surgery; Immobilization

- Acute, initial therapy (usually *Staphylococcus*, streptococci, *Haemophilus*) | Infants: cefuroxime or cefotaxime 100-150 mg/kg/day IV, IM div q8h; Children > 4 yrs: nafcillin 150 mg/kg/day IV, div q6h x 3 weeks or longer. Alternatives: other beta-lactams, clindamycin | In children add ceftazidime to nafcillin if Gram-negative rods in pus, pending culture and susceptibility results

- Acute, other organisms | See Section VII for preferred antibiotics |

- *Pseudomonas aeruginosa* | Ceftazidime 150 mg/kg/day IV, IM div q8h OR mezlocillin or ticarcillin 200-300 mg/kg/day IV div q6h AND (compromised host) gentamicin 6 mg/kg/day IM, IV or amikacin 15-20 mg/kg/day IM, IV div q8h; x 10 days | If thorough surgical debridement not done, longer therapy required

- Chronic (staphylococcal) | Dicloxacillin 75-100 mg/kg/day PO div q6h OR cephradine/cephalexin 100-150 mg/kg/day PO div q6h; x 6-12 months | Surgery; Monitor serum for bactericidal titer or antibiotic concentration (See Section IV for details)

C. EYE INFECTIONS

Hordeolum (sty) or chalazion | None (Topical antibiotic not necessary) | Warm compresses; I & D when necessary

Acute conjunctivitis | Polymyxin B-bacitracin or sulfacetamide ophthalmic drops q2h or ointment q4-6h | See page 9 for chlamydial, gonococcal, pseudomonal infection

Herpetic conjunctivitis | Trifluoridine sol'n 1 drop q2-3h while awake x 7-14 days; OR vidarabine ointment topically q3h until 1 week after healing | Consider steroids if keratitis present (refer to ophthalmologist)

21

Clinical Diagnosis	Therapy	Comments
Periorbital cellulitis (Pre-septal infection) - Associated with sinusitis	Cefuroxime or ceftriaxone 100-150 mg/kg/day IV, IM div q 8h x 5-7 days	Follow with oral antibiotic (See page 25)
- Idiopathic (*Haemophilus* or pneumococcal)	Cefuroxime or ceftriaxone 100-150 mg/kg/day IV, IM div q8h <u>OR</u> chloramphenicol 50-75 mg/kg/day IV, PO div q6h; x 7-10 days	Lumbar puncture to R/O meningitis; LARGER DOSAGES NEEDED FOR MENINGITIS
- Associated with periorbital skin lesion (streptococcal, staphylococcal)	Nafcillin 150 mg/kg/day IV div q6h x 7-10 days	Oral antistaphylococcal antibiotic for less severe infection
Orbital cellulitis (Post-septal infection)	Nafcillin 150 mg/kg/day IV div q6h <u>AND</u> chloramphenicol 75-100 mg/kg/day IV, PO div q6h x 10-14 days	Usually staphylococcal or Gram-negative bacilli; Surgical drainage of pus
Dacryocystitis	No antibiotic usually; when needed, based on Gram stain and culture of pus	Warm compresses; May require surgical probing of naso-lachrymal duct
Endophthalmitis		NOTE: Subconjunctival/sub-tenon antibiotic often needed; steroids commonly used
- Staphylococcal	Nafcillin 150 mg/kg/day IV div q6h x 10-14 days; Alternatives: other beta-lactams or vancomycin	Penicillin for susceptible organisms
- Pneumococcal, meningococcal	Penicillin G 250,000 u/kg/day IV div q4h x 10-14 days (chloramphenicol or vancomycin for penicillin-resistant pneumococci)	R/O meningitis

22

- Gonococcal	Ceftriaxone 50 mg/kg once daily IV, IM x 7 days or longer
- *Pseudomonas*	Mezlocillin or ticarcillin 200-300 mg/kg/day IV div q4-6h AND gentamicin 6 mg/kg/day IM, IV or amikacin 15-20 mg/kg/day IM, IV div q6h x 10-14 days	Piperacillin or ceftazidime are alternatives

Retinitis

- Cytomegalovirus	Ganciclovir OR foscarnet (for dosage see Section X)

D. EAR AND SINUS INFECTIONS

External otitis, bacterial	Optimal therapy unknown; cleaning canal of detritus important; antibiotic or antibiotic-steroid drops (e.g. Cortisporin suspension) customarily used but efficacy not proved	Wick moistened with Burow's sol'n used for marked swelling of canal; For "swimmer's ear", VoSol or alcohol-vinegar mixture to canal after water exposure
External otitis, fungal (otomycosis)	Topical 1/2 alcohol - 1/2 vinegar sol'n OR 25% M-cresyl acetate (Cresylate) t.i.d.	Usually *Aspergillus*; Debride canal
Furuncle of external canal	Cefadroxil 30 mg/kg/day div q12h OR cloxacillin 50 mg/kg/day div q6-8h OR cephradine/cephalexin 50 mg/kg/day div q6-8h	I & D; Antibiotic not necessary unless cellulitis
Bullous myringitis	Antibiotics, as for otitis media with effusion (see below)	Current concept is that this is simply one manifestation of acute otitis media

23

Clinical Diagnosis	Therapy	Comments
Otitis media, acute with effusion		
- Newborns	See Section V	Gram stain and culture of pus if spontaneous rupture; IF prior antibiotic therapy or compromised host, suspect unusual infection and do tympanocentesis for culture; Effective oral therapy for beta-lactam resistant pneumococci not established
- Infants and children (pneumococcus, *Haemophilus*, *Moraxella* most common)	Amoxicillin or Augmentin 40 mg/kg/day PO div q8h; OR erythromycin-sulfa combination 40 mg/kg/day of erythro component PO div q6-8h OR cefaclor 40 mg/kg/day PO div q8-12h OR TMP/SMX 8 mg/kg/day of TMP component PO div q12h OR cefixime 8 mg/kg once daily or div q12h; x 5-10 days OR cefprozil or loracarbef 30 mg/kg/day div q12h OR cefpodoxime 10 mg/kg/day div q12h OR ceftibuten 9 mg/kg once daily OR clarithromycin 15 mg/kg/day div q12h	

A Note on Acute Otitis Media with Effusion: There are several effective antibiotic regimens for management of AOM. Customarily amoxicillin is used initially and other drugs are given for amoxicillin failures or relapses. The physician should consider advantages and disadvantages regarding antibacterial spectrum, palatability of suspensions, and cost. TMP/SMX is not effective for Group A streptococcal infection. When prophylaxis is indicated, use amoxicillin or sulfa drug in one-half the therapeutic dose once or twice daily.

Clinical Diagnosis	Therapy	Comments
Mastoiditis, acute (pneumococcus, staphylococcus, Gr. A streptococcus; *Haemophilus* rare)	Nafcillin 150 mg/kg/day IV div q6h OR cefuroxime 100-150 mg/kg/day IV, IM div q8h x 10 days; Alternatives: other beta-lactams or vancomycin for penicillin-resistant pneumococci	R/O meningitis; Surgery as needed; Change to oral therapy after clinical improvement
Mastoiditis, chronic	Antibiotics only for acute superinfections (according to culture of drainage); also, when chronic *Pseudomonas* infection, mezlocillin or ticarcillin 200-300	Daily cleansing of ear important; After resolution, use amoxicillin or sulfa prophylaxis for otitis; If

24

Sinusitis, acute (*Haemophilus*, pneumococcus, streptococcus, *Moraxella*)

Same as for acute otitis media but 14-21 days may be needed

Sinus irrigations when indicated

E. NOSE AND THROAT INFECTIONS

Diphtheria

Penicillin G 150,000 u/kg/day IV div q6h OR erythromycin 40-50 mg/kg/day PO x 14 days

Plus antitoxin; Isolation until 3 daily nose and throat cultures negative

Streptococcal tonsillopharyngitis, scarlet fever and peritonsillar cellulitis

Penicillin V 25-50 mg/kg/day PO div q6-8h x 10 days OR benzathine penicillin 25,000 u/kg IM (max 1.2 million u) as a single dose; Alternatives: oral cephalosporins

Erythromycin or clindamycin for penicillin-allergic patients (Caution:~5% of Group A strep resistant)

Epiglottitis (aryepiglottitis, supraglottitis) or **bacterial tracheitis**

Cefuroxime 100-150 mg/kg/day IV, IM div q8h OR chloramphenicol 50-75 mg/kg/day IV div q6h x 5-7 days; Alternatives: cefotaxime, ceftriaxone

Provide airway; Almost always caused by *Haemophilus influenzae*, type b (epiglottitis) or Gram-positive cocci (tracheitis)

Retropharyngeal or lateral pharyngeal cellulitis or abscess

Clindamycin 30 mg/kg/day PO, IV, IM div q6h OR nafcillin 150 mg/kg/day IV div q6h and chloramphenicol 50-75 mg/kg/day IV, PO

Usually aerobes and anaerobes; I & D when pus present; Consider tonsillectomy for peritonsillar abscess

F. LOWER RESPIRATORY INFECTIONS

Respiratory syncytial virus infection (bronchiolitis, pneumonia)

Ribavirin 6 g vial (20 mg/ml in sterile water) aerosolized by SPAG-2 over 18-20 hr period daily x 3-5 days

Treat only for severe disease or patients with underlying cardiopulmonary disease

Clinical Diagnosis	Therapy	Comments
Pertussis	Erythromycin (estolate may be preferable) 50 mg/kg/day PO div q6h x 10 days (re-administer vomited doses, or change to ampicillin 100 mg/kg/day IV, IM div q6h)	Hospitalize young babies; Avoid mist therapy; Avoid cough suppressants; Isolate until 2 daily cultures negative or for 10 days
Tuberculosis		
- Primary	Isoniazid 10 mg/kg/day (max 300 mg) PO, IM x 9 mos AND rifampin 10-15 mg/kg/day (max 600 mg) PO, IV x 9 mos AND pyrazinamide 25 mg/kg/day PO x 2 mos; If in area with known drug resistance, add ethambutol 20 mg/kg/day PO OR streptomycin 30 mg/kg/day IM initially	Test for HIV infection; Two drug regimen with isoniazid and rifampin satisfactory if TB strain known to be susceptible to both drugs; For drug resistant strains, obtain consultation with Health Department
- Skin test conversion	Isoniazid 10-15 mg/kg/day (max 300 mg) PO daily x 9 months	Single drug Rx if no clinical or radiographic evidence of disease
- Exposed infant < 6 yrs, or immunocompromised patient	Isoniazid 10-15 mg/kg PO daily x 3 mos after last exposure	If PPD remains negative and child well, stop prophylaxis
Lung abscess		
- Primary, putrid (i.e., foul-smelling)	Clindamycin 30 mg/kg/day PO, IM, IV div q6-8h; OR penicillin G 100,000 u/kg/day IV div q4-6h and chloramphenicol 50-75 mg/kg/day IV, PO div q6h; x 10 days or longer	Usually polymicrobial infection with aerobes and anaerobes

Condition	Treatment	Comments
- Primary, non-putrid	Cefuroxime 100-150 mg/kg/day IV, IM div q8h or other beta-lactamase-resistant beta-lactam; x 10 days or longer	Bronchoscopy necessary if abscess fails to drain; Surgical excision rarely necessary
- Secondary to other focus of infection (osteomyelitis, etc.)	Nafcillin 150 mg/kg/day IV div q6h x 10 days or longer OR other beta-lactams	Usually staphylococcal; cephalosporin for coliforms
Pneumonia in immunosuppressed, neutropenic host	Nafcillin 150 mg/kg/day IV div q6h or vancomycin 40 mg/kg/day IV div q6h (if methicillin-resistant Staph suspected) AND ceftazidime 150 mg/kg/day IV div q8h; Alternative: mezlocillin or ticarcillin 200-300 mg/kg/day IV div q6h AND amikacin 15-22.5 mg/kg/day or gentamicin 6 mg/kg/day IM, IV div q8h AND nafcillin (as above)	Consider opportunist bacteria, pneumocystis, cytomegalovirus, fungi, tuberculosis; Biopsy or bronchoalveolar lavage of lung may be needed to establish diagnosis
Acute pulmonary exacerbations of cystic fibrosis	Ticarcillin 300-400 mg/kg/day IV div q4h AND tobramycin 6-10 mg/kg/day IM, IV div q6-8h; Alternatives: other anti-*Pseudomonas* beta-lactams and aminoglycosides OR ceftazidime 150 mg/kg/day IV div q8h; x 7-10 days OR aztreonam 200 mg/kg/day IV div q6h	Larger than normal dosages of aminoglycosides required in most patients with cystic fibrosis; Monitor peak serum concentrations of aminoglycosides
Pneumocystis carinii pneumonia	(See page 56)	
Bronchitis, acute	No antibiotic for most cases (viral); if bacterial infection suspected, use same drugs as for acute otitis or sinusitis (page 24)	*Haemophilus, Moraxella,* pneumococcus most common pathogens in adults and (?) in children

27

Clinical Diagnosis	Therapy	Comments
Allergic bronchopulmonary aspergillosis	Prednisone 0.5 mg/kg every other day	Larger dosages may lead to tissue invasion
Pneumonia with empyema		Initial therapy based on Gram stain of empyema fluid
- Pneumococcal, Group A streptococcal	Penicillin G 150,000 u/kg/day IV div q4-6h x 10 days (Change to PO penicillin V in same dosage after clinical improvement); Alternatives: cephalosporins, clindamycin	Closed chest tube drainage of purulent fluid; Vancomycin for penicillin-resistant pneumococci
- Staphylococcal	Nafcillin 150 mg/kg/day IV div q6h <u>OR</u> vancomycin 40 mg/kg/day div q6h x 21 days or longer (Alternatives: cephalosporins)	Closed chest tube drainage of empyema
- *Haemophilus influenzae* b or pneumonia of unestablished etiology (< 5 yrs of age)	Cefuroxime or cefotaxime 100-150 mg/kg/day IV, IM div q8h; <u>OR</u> ampicillin 150 mg/kg/day IV, IM div q6h <u>AND</u> chloramphenicol 50-75 mg/kg/day IV, PO div q6h x 10-14 days; <u>OR</u> ceftriaxone 50 mg/kg IV, IM once daily	Closed chest tube drainage; R/O meningitis; LARGER DOSAGES NEEDED FOR MENINGITIS
Lobar or segmental consolidation		
- *Haemophilus*, or unknown etiology	Cefuroxime 100-150 mg/kg/day IV, IM div q8h x 10 days	Change to PO after improvement
- Pneumococcal	Penicillin G 150,000 u/kg/day IV div q4-6h x 10 days; Vancomycin for penicillin-resistant strains	Change to PO penicillin V in same dosage after improvement

Klebsiella pneumoniae | Gentamicin 6 mg/kg/day IM, IV div q8h x 10 days or longer OR amikacin 15-20 mg/kg/day IM, IV div q8h; (Alternative: cefotaxime 150 mg/kg/day IV, IM div q8h) | Suspect if distended lobe; Abscesses common but empyema rare

Bronchopneumonia

- Mild to moderate illness | No antibiotic therapy unless epidemiological/clinical reasons to suspect specific pathogen other than virus | Most viral; Broad spectrum antibiotics increase risk of superinfection

- Serious, life-threatening illness | Initially, until etiology established, nafcillin 150 mg/kg/day IV div q6h AND gentamicin 6 mg/kg/day or amikacin 15-22.5 mg/kg/day IM, IV div q8h (Cefotaxime or cefuroxime may be effective) | Consider needle aspiration of lung to establish diagnosis (Gram stain and culture of aspirate); Tracheal aspirate Gram stain and culture may be helpful

Afebrile pneumonia syndrome of early infancy | Supportive, or (if chlamydia suspected) erythromycin 40 mg/kg/day PO div q6h x 14 days | Most viral or chlamydial; Often interstitial infiltrate

Other pneumonias of established etiology

- *Chlamydia pneumoniae* (TWAR), *C. psittaci* or *C. trachomatis* | A macrolide OR tetracycline (pts >7 yrs) (Ampicillin for *C. trachomatis*) | For dosage see Section X

- Cytomegalovirus | Ganciclovir (plus IV immune globulin) | For dosage see Section X

- *E. coli, Enterobacter* spp. | An aminoglycoside or cephalosporin | For dosage see Section X

- *Francisella tularensis* | Gentamicin or streptomycin | See page 42

- Fungi | Amphotericin B or combined therapy | For dosage see Section VIII

Clinical Diagnosis	Therapy	Comments
- Influenza A	Amantadine	For dosage, see page 40
- Legionnaires' disease	A macrolide and rifampin	For dosage, see Section X
- Melioidosis	See page 41	
- *Mycoplasma pneumoniae*	A macrolide or tetracycline	For dosage, see Section X
- *Paragonimus westermani*	Praziquantel	For dosage, see page 61
- *Pseudomonas aeruginosa*	Anti-*Pseudomonas* penicillin AND amino-glycoside; OR ceftazidime	For dosage, see Section X

G. HEART INFECTIONS

Purulent pericarditis

		SURGICAL DRAINAGE OF PUS
- *Staphylococcus aureus*	Nafcillin 150 mg/kg/day IV div q6h OR (for methicillin-resistant staphylococci) vancomycin 40 mg/kg/day IV div q6h x 3 wks or longer	Change to penicillin G if susceptible
- *Haemophilus influenzae* b	Cefuroxime 100-150 mg/kg/day IV, IM div q8h x 10-14 days; Alternatives: cefotaxime, ceftriaxone	Ampicillin for beta-lactamase-negative strains
- Pneumococcus, meningococcus, Group A streptococcus	Penicillin G 150,000 u/kg/day IV, IM div q4-6h x 10-14 days	Vancomycin for penicillin-resistant pneumococci
- Coliform bacilli	Cefotaxime 100-150 mg/kg/day IV, IM div q6-8h x 3 wks or longer; Alternatives: other cephalosporins, aminoglycoside	Alternative drugs depending on susceptibilities
- Tuberculous	(See page 26)	Corticosteroids for first

30

Endocarditis

- Viridans streptococcus	Penicillin G 150,000 u/kg/day IV div q4-6h x 30 days (optional: AND streptomycin 30 mg/kg/day IM div q12h during first 14 days); OR vancomycin 40 mg/kg/day IV div q6h	Monitor serum bactericidal activity; See Section IV for discussion of oral therapy
- Enterococcus	Ampicillin 150 mg/kg/day IV, IM div q6h x 30 days AND gentamicin 6 mg/kg/day IM, IV div q8h OR penicillin G 250,000 u/kg/day IV div q4-6h AND streptomycin 30 mg/kg/day IM div q12h; x 30 days	Longest experience with the penicillin-streptomycin regimen; Combined Rx used for synergistic bactericidal activity
- *Staphylococcus aureus*, *Staphylococcus epidermidis*	Nafcillin 150 mg/kg/day IV div q6h x 6 wks OR, for methicillin-resistant staphylococci, vancomycin 40 mg/kg/day IV div q6h; Consider adding rifampin or aminoglycoside for synergistic effect	Surgery may be necessary in acute phase; Avoid cephalo-sporins because of conflicting data on efficacy
- Pneumococcus, gonococcus, Group A streptococcus	Penicillin G 150,000 u/kg/day IV div q4-6h x 30 days (vancomycin for penicillin-resistant pneumococci)	Ceftriaxone for gonococcus until susceptibilities known
- Prophylaxis for:		**If penicillin allergy:**
- Dental and upper respiratory procedures	Amoxicillin PO 50 mg/kg 1 hr before procedure and 25 mg/kg 6 hr later OR Ampicillin IM, IV 50 mg/kg 30 min before AND gentamicin IM, IV 2 mg/kg 30 min before	Erythromycin 20 mg/kg 2 hr before and 10 mg/kg 6 hr later Vancomycin IV 20 mg/kg during 1 hr before procedure
- Genitourinary and gastrointestinal procedures	Ampicillin IM, IV AND gentamicin IM, IV (as above); repeat 8 hrs later	Vancomycin IV (as above) AND gentamicin IM, IV (as above)

31

Clinical Diagnosis	Therapy	Comments
H. GASTROINTESTINAL INFECTIONS	(See Section IX for parasitic infections)	
Shigellosis	Trimethoprim/sulfamethoxazole 10 mg TMP-50 mg SMX/kg/day PO, IV div q12h x 5 days OR (for susceptible strains) ampicillin 100 mg/kg/day IV, IM, PO div q6h	Tetracycline, chloramphenicol, absorbable sulfas, nalidixic acid also effective when *Shigella* susceptible; Avoid anti-peristaltic drugs
Salmonellosis	None for usual self-limited diarrhea OR amoxicillin 50 mg/kg/day PO div q8h x 5-7 days OR TMP/SMX as for shigellosis (For typhoid fever see page 43)	Treat infants with bacteremia, compromised hosts and those with septic clinical picture or colitis (IV antibiotics for bacteremia)
Escherichia coli		
- Enteropathogenic	Neomycin 100 mg/kg/day PO div q6-8h	Most traditional "entero-pathogenic" strains not toxigenic or invasive
- Enterotoxigenic	Trimethoprim-sulfamethoxazole (as for shigellosis) OR neomycin or colistin PO	Most illnesses brief and self-limited
- Enteroinvasive	(?) Orally absorbable antibiotic, such as ampicillin, amoxicillin or trimethoprim-sulfamethoxazole	No controlled clinical trials on which to base a recommendation
"Turista" (traveler's diarrhea)	As for enterotoxigenic *E. coli* above	50-75% of cases due to toxi-genic *E. coli*; If not improved after 5 days, investigate for *Shigella, Giardia*, etc.

Yersinia enterocolitica	Antimicrobial therapy probably not of value	May mimic appendicitis
Campylobacter jejuni	Erythromycin 40 mg/kg/day PO div q6h x 5 days	Abdominal pain may mimic acute surgical abdomen
Aeromonas sp.	(?) Trimethoprim-sulfamethoxazole as for shigellosis	Efficacy not established
Antibiotic-associated colitis	Vancomycin 50 mg/kg/day PO div q6h x 7 days; Alternatives: metronidazole 20 mg/kg/day PO div q6h; bacitracin 2000 u/kg/day PO div q6h	Due to overgrowth of *Cl. difficile* in gut; Vancomycin may cause emergence of resistant enterococci in gut
Perirectal abscess	Clindamycin 30-40 mg/kg/day IV, PO div q6-8h AND aminoglycoside or cephalosporin	*S. aureus* common but may be mixed with coliforms, anaerobes; Surgical drainage

I. GENITOURINARY AND SEXUALLY TRANSMITTED INFECTIONS

Genital herpes infection	Acyclovir 400 mg PO 3 x daily OR acyclovir 200 mg PO 5 x daily x 7-10 days OR (for severe disease) acyclovir 15 mg/kg/day as 1 hr IV infusion div q8h x 5-7 days	Most effective when started early in course of infection; For prevention of recurrence 400 mg 2 x daily

CONSIDER TESTING FOR HIV INFECTION IN CHILDREN WITH SEXUALLY TRANSMITTED DISEASES

33

Clinical Diagnosis	Therapy	Comments
Urinary tract infection		
- Acute cystitis	Sulfisoxazole 120-150 mg/kg/day PO div q6h <u>OR</u> amoxicillin 30 mg/kg/day div q6-8h x 7-10 days; For recurrent infections, trimethoprim-sulfamethoxazole 8 mg TMP-40 mg SMX/kg/day div q12h	"*In vivo*" susceptibility test: follow-up culture after 36-48 hrs treatment. If culture positive, change treatment according to *in vitro* susceptibilities
- Acute pyelonephritis	Gentamicin 6 mg/kg/day IV, IM div q8h <u>OR</u> trimethoprim-sulfamethoxazole 8 mg TMP-40 mg SMX/kg/day PO, IV div q12h x 10 days	Parenteral drug if sepsis suspected; Change to appropriate oral drug after clinical response
- Prophylaxis for recurrent bacteriuria	Trimethoprim-sulfamethoxazole 2 mg TMP-10 mg SMX/kg PO q1-2 days <u>OR</u> nitrofurantoin 1-2 mg/kg PO q1-2 days at bedtime	Prophylaxis for patients with reflux or frequent infections
Epididymitis	Cefuroxime 100-150 mg/kg/day div q8h <u>OR</u> nafcillin 150 mg/kg/day IV div q6h and chloramphenicol 50-75 mg/kg/day IV, PO div q6h; x 7-10 days	Usually due to *Haemophilus* or *S. aureus* in young children; Treat as for gonorrhea and chlamydia in older children
Trichomoniasis	See Section IX	
Vaginitis or cervicitis		
- Vulvovaginal candidiasis	See Section VIII	
- *Shigella*	As for diarrhea (see page 32)	50% have bloody discharge; Usually not associated with diarrhea

34

Condition	Treatment	Comments
- Chlamydial	Doxycycline 4 mg/kg/day (max. 200 mg) PO div q12h OR erythromycin 40 mg/kg/day PO div q6h x 7 days	*Chlamydia* occurs in pre-pubertal as well as post-pubertal children
- Bacterial vaginosis (formerly "nonspecific vaginitis")	Metronidazole 15-20 mg/kg/day PO div q8h x 7 days OR clindamycin 20 mg/kg/day PO div q12h x 7 days	Caused by synergy of *Gardnerella* with anaerobes
Gonorrhea		
- Newborns	See Section V	
- Genital infections	Treatment regimens of demonstrated efficacy for children: 1) Ceftriaxone 250 IM as single dose 2) Procaine penicillin G 100,000 u/kg IM as single dose (2 injection sites) AND probenecid 25 mg/kg PO (max 1 g) 3) Amoxicillin 50 mg/kg PO as single dose AND probenecid 25 mg/kg PO 4) Spectinomycin 40 mg/kg IM as single dose 5) Cefuroxime 25 mg/kg IM as single dose	Ceftriaxone preferred; Serologic test for syphilis; Repeat in 3 mos. if treated with something other than penicillin; Social evaluation re possibility of child abuse; Follow with treatment for presumed chlamydia
- Disseminated gonococcal infection	Ceftriaxone 50 mg/kg/day IM, IV once daily OR cefotaxime IV div q8h; x 7 days	No controlled studies in children; Increase dosage for meningitis
Syphilis		See most recent CDC <u>Sexually Transmitted Diseases Treatment Guidelines</u>
- Congenital	See Section V	

35

Clinical Diagnosis	Therapy	Comments
- Primary, secondary	Benzathine penicillin G 2,400,000 u IM (approximately 50,000 u/kg) in 2 injection sites OR doxycycline 4 mg/kg/day (max 200 mg) PO div q12h x 14 days OR erythromycin 2 g/day PO div q6h x 14 days	Follow-up serologic tests at 3, 6 and 12 months; Do not use benzathine-procaine penicillin mixtures
- Syphilis of more than 1 year duration	Benzathine penicillin G 2,400,000 u IM (50,000 u/kg) in 2 injection sites weekly for 3 doses OR procaine penicillin 2,400,000 u IM daily plus probenecid 500 mg PO div q6h x 10-14 days	Optimal treatment schedule not established
Chancroid	Ceftriaxone 250 mg IM as single dose OR erythromycin 2 g/day PO div q6h x 7 days OR azithromycin 1 g PO as single dose	Serologic test for syphilis
Lymphogranuloma venereum (*Chlamydia trachomatis*)	Doxycycline 4 mg/kg/day (max 200 mg) PO div q12h OR erythromycin 2 g/day PO div q6h x 21 days	
Pelvic inflammatory disease	Cefoxitin 2 g IV q6h AND doxycycline 100 mg PO bid OR clindamycin 900 mg IV q8h OR ceftriaxone 250 mg IM once followed by doxycycline (as above)	Two drugs given until clinical improvement and followed by doxycycline alone to complete 10-14 days

36

J. CENTRAL NERVOUS SYSTEM INFECTIONS

Bacterial meningitis

NOTE: Dexamethasone (0.6 mg/kg/day IV div q6h x 4 days) as an adjunct to antibiotic therapy decreases hearing deficits and possibly other neurologic sequelae in *Haemophilus* meningitis and possibly other types. The first dose of dexamethasone is preferably given before the first dose of antibiotic.

- Neonatal

See Section V

- *Haemophilus influenzae* b

Cefotaxime 200 mg/kg/day IV div q6-8h OR ceftriaxone either 100 mg/kg/day IV div q12h or 80 mg/kg IV, IM once daily
Alternative: Ampicillin 200-400 mg/kg/day IV div q6h AND chloramphenicol 100 mg/kg/day IV div q6h; x 10 days

Chloramphenicol can be given PO; Rifampin prophylaxis for patients and contacts according to Red Book recommendations

- Pneumococcus

Penicillin G 250,000 u/kg/day IV div q4h x 10 days; For penicillin-insensitive pneumococci use chloramphenicol 100 mg/kg/day IV, div q6h; For penicillin-resistant pneumococci use vancomycin 60 mg/kg/day IV div q6h (?) plus rifampin 20 mg/kg/day IV

Some of pneumococci relatively resistant ("insensitive") or frankly resistant to penicillin; Some of the latter are also resistant to cephalosporins

- Meningococcus
  (Including meningococcemia)

Penicillin G 250,000 u/kg/day IV div q4h x 7 days; Regimens given for *Haemophilus* are effective for meningococcal infection; Rare strains are resistant to penicillin

Meningococcal prophylaxis: rifampin 10 mg/kg PO q12h x 4 doses; Trisulfapyrimidines 25 mg/kg PO q12h x 4 doses if organism from index case susceptible

37

Clinical Diagnosis	Therapy	Comments
- Unknown bacterial, 1-3 mos of age	Ampicillin (as above) AND cefotaxime 200 mg/kg/day IV div q6h	Both "neonatal" and "infant" pathogens encountered in this age group
- Unknown bacterial, after 3 mos of age	As for Haemophilus (above)	
- Tuberculous	Isoniazid 15 mg/kg/day PO, IM div q12-24h AND rifampin 15 mg/kg/day, IV, PO div q12-24h x 12 mos AND streptomycin 30 mg/kg/day IM div q12h for first 4 weeks of therapy AND pyrazinamide 30 mg/kg/day PO div q12-24h for first 2 months	Hyponatremia from inappropriate ADH common; Ventricular drainage may be necessary; Steroids suppress symptoms and may improve prognosis
Shunt infections		
- S. epidermidis or S. aureus	Vancomycin 60 mg/kg/day IV div q6h OR nafcillin 150 mg/kg/day (?) PLUS an aminoglycoside or rifampin; x 10-14 days	Surgery for shunt revision usually necessary; May be synergy between antibiotics
- Coliform bacilli	Cefotaxime 200 mg/kg/day IV div q6h OR ampicillin 200 mg/kg/day IV div q6h AND gentamicin 6 mg/kg/day or amikacin 15-20 mg/kg/day IV, IM div q8h; x 21 days or longer	Select appropriate drug based on in vitro susceptibilities

Brain abscess — Until etiology established nafcillin or vancomycin (as for meningitis) AND cefotaxime (as for meningitis) AND metronidazole 30 mg/kg/day IV, PO div q8h; x 7-10 days after surgery; Longer therapy if no surgery — Surgery; Anaerobes common; Add anti-*Pseudomonas* drug if secondary to chronic otitis; Follow abscess size with CT scans

Herpes simplex encephalitis — Acyclovir 30 mg/kg/day as 1 hr or longer IV infusion div q8h OR vidarabine 15 mg/kg as 12 hr or longer IV infusion daily x 10 days — Larger dosages and longer durations of acyclovir therapy are being tested

Toxoplasma encephalitis — See Section IX

K. MISCELLANEOUS SYSTEMIC INFECTIONS

Acquired immunodeficiency syndrome — See HIV infection below

Actinomycosis — Penicillin G 250,000 u/kg/day IV div q4h until improved; thereafter penicillin V 100 mg/kg/day PO div q6h x several months — Surgery as indicated; Tetracycline for penicillin-allergic

Brucellosis — Tetracycline 40 mg/kg/day PO, IV div q6h (IV daily dose should not exceed 2 g) if > 7 yrs; TMP 10 mg/kg-SMX 50 mg/kg/day div q12h if <7 yrs; Rifampin (15-20 mg/kg/day div q12h) given as second drug; x 6 weeks or longer — Add gentamicin 5-6 mg/kg/day IV, IM div q8h for the first 5 days

Cat-scratch disease — Supportive; aspiration of pus — Aminoglycoside, rifampin, ciprofloxacin may be effective

Chickenpox — Acyclovir 40-80 mg/kg/day PO div q6h x 5-7 days, when indicated (Most cases do not require therapy — Parenteral therapy for severe cases (See Varicella-zoster, disseminated, page 43)

39

Clinical Diagnosis	Therapy	Comments
Ehrlichiosis	(See Rickettsial infection on page 42)	
Febrile neutropenic patient	Nafcillin (or vancomycin if methicillin-resistant Staph is suspected) <u>AND</u> anti-*Pseudomonas* beta-lactam <u>AND</u> aminoglycoside; <u>OR</u> anti-staphylococcal drug <u>AND</u> ceftazidime	If no response in 5-7 days and no bacterial etiology demonstrated, consider empiric antifungal therapy with amphotericin B; Dosages in Section X
Human immunodeficiency virus infection	Zidovudine 720 mg/m^2/day PO div q6h (max 200 mg per dose)	Didanosine and zalcitabine also used
Infant botulism	No antibiotic or antitoxin; aminoglycosides potentiate effect of toxin; (trivalent antitoxin for food-borne or wound botulism)	ICU supportive therapy; Enemas to remove constipated stool and toxin is controversial
Influenza A infection	Amantadine 5 mg/kg/day (max. 200 mg) PO div q12h x 7 days; Ribavirin aerosol (as for RSV infection, page 25) may be effective	Treat within 48-72 hrs of onset; Rx especially for high-risk patients
Kawasaki syndrome	No antibiotics; IV gamma globulin 2 g/kg as single dose	Aspirin qs to achieve serum conc of 20-30 mg/dl in acute phase; prolonged low dosage (3-5 mg/kg/day) aspirin Rx may decrease risk of coronary artery disease
Leprosy	Dapsone 1 mg/kg PO daily <u>PLUS</u> clofazimine 1 mg/kg PO daily <u>PLUS</u> rifampin 10 mg/kg PO once monthly	Clofazimine necessary because of increased resistance to dapsone

Disease	Treatment	Notes
Leptospirosis	Penicillin G 250,000 u/kg/day IV, IM div q4-6h OR tetracycline 40 mg/kg/day PO div q6h; x 7-10 days	
Lyme disease	Early disease: Doxycycline 4 mg/kg/day PO div q12h (pts >7 yrs) OR amoxicillin 40 mg/kg/day (max 3 g) (?) with probenecid 25 mg/kg/day (max 1500) PO div q8h; x 21 days	Late disease: ceftriaxone 100 (CNS) or 50 (others) mg/kg once daily IM, IV x 14-21 days
Measles	Supportive therapy; Ribavirin has been used 15 mg/kg/day IV div q8h x 10 days (double dose on 1st day); Vitamin A therapy reported to be beneficial in malnourished	Consider ribavirin in severe disease/compromised host (IV formulation not commercially available)
Melioidosis	Acute sepsis: Ceftazidime 120 mg/kg/day IV div q8h OR chloramphenicol 50-75 mg/kg/day IV, PO div q6h AND sulfisoxazole 120-150 mg PO div q6h AND an aminoglycoside; x 10-14 days Chronic infection: Trimethoprim-sulfamethoxazole 8 mg TMP/kg-40 mg SMX/kg/day div q12h x several weeks	Ceftazidime more effective than conventional 3 drug therapy in one study Tetracycline for children > 7 years of age
Mycobacteriosis (Disseminated MAI disease in compromised host)	Usually treated with 4 or 5 drugs; e.g. ciprofloxacin, clofazimine, ethambutol, rifampin, amikacin	See Section X for dosage
Nocardiosis	Sulfisoxazole 120-150 mg/kg/day PO div q6h x 6 weeks or longer; For severe infection, amikacin 15-20 mg/kg/day IM, IV div q8h	Surgery when indicated; Trimethoprim-sulfamethoxazole or cycloserine as alternatives

Clinical Diagnosis	Therapy	Comments
Peritonitis		
- Primary	Penicillin G 150,000 u/kg/day IV div q4h x 7-10 days	Usually pneumococcal; Other antibiotics according to culture and susceptibility tests
- Secondary to bowel perforation or appendicitis	Clindamycin 30 mg/kg/day IV, IM div q6h AND gentamicin 6 mg/kg/day IV, IM div q8h x 10 days or longer	Many other regimens claimed to be effective; Add ampicillin for enterococcus
- Secondary to peritoneal dialysis	Antibiotic added to dialysate in concentrations approximating those attained in serum for systemic disease (e.g. 8 mcg/ml for gentamicin; 50 mcg/ml for vancomycin, etc.)	Selection of antibiotic based on organism isolated from peritoneal fluid; Systemic antibiotics if there is accompanying bacteremia
Rickettsial infection	Tetracycline (Pts >7 yrs) 40 mg/kg/day PO div q6h (Initially can be given IV) OR chloramphenicol 50-75 mg/kg/day IV, PO div q6h; x 10-14 days	Chloramphenicol is preferred for young children
Tetanus	Penicillin G 100,000 u/kg/day IV div q4-6h x 10 days	Plus antitoxin and sedation
Toxic shock syndrome	Nafcillin 150 mg/kg/day IV div q6h x 7 days	General supportive care of prime importance
Tularemia	Gentamicin 6 mg/kg/day IM, IV div q8h OR streptomycin 30 mg/kg/day IM div q12h; x 7-10 days (Dosage of streptomycin may be reduced by 1/2 after 3 days)	Tetracycline less effective alternative

42

Typhoid fever	Chloramphenicol 50(PO)-75(IV) mg/kg/day div q6h OR amoxicillin 100 mg/kg/day PO div q8h x 14 days	TMP/SMX; Ceftriaxone and cefotaxime are also effective
Varicella-zoster, disseminated (compromised host)	Acyclovir 1500 mg/m²/day (approx 45 mg/kg/day) IV as 1-2 hr infusion div q8h OR vidarabine 10 mg/kg/day as 6 hr IV infusion; x 5 days	Also used for severe or complicated chickenpox

43

VII. PREFERRED THERAPY FOR SPECIFIC PATHOGENS

NOTES: 1. For parasitic and fungal infections see Sections IX and VIII, respectively.
2. Limitations of space do not permit listing of all possible alternative antimicrobials.

Organism	Clinical Illness	Drug of Choice	Alternatives
Acinetobacter baumanii	Sepsis, meningitis	Imipenem	Anti-*Pseudomonas* beta-lactam + amikacin; TMP/SMX
Actinobacillus actinomycetemcomitans	Abscesses, endocarditis	Ampicillin	Tetracycline (Pts >7 yrs); chloramphenicol
Actinomyces israelii	Actinomycosis	Penicillin G	Tetracycline (Pts >7 yrs); ampicillin
Aeromonas spp.	Diarrhea, sepsis, cellulitis	TMP/SMX	An aminoglycoside; imipenem
Afipia felis	(?) Cat-scratch disease	(?) Aminoglycoside	(?) rifampin; ciprofloxacin
Arcanobacterium haemolyticum	Pharyngitis	A macrolide	Penicillin G; a cephalosporin
Bacillus anthracis	Anthrax	Penicillin G	A macrolide; tetracycline (Pts >7 yrs)
Bacteroides fragilis	Peritonitis, sepsis, abscesses	Chloramphenicol; clindamycin; metronidazole for CNS infection	Cefoxitin; anti-*Pseudomonas* penicillins; imipenem
Bacteroides, other spp.	Pneumonia, sepsis, abscesses	Penicillin G	Ampicillin; clindamycin; chloramphenicol; metronidazole

44

		(Pts >7 yrs)	
Bordetella spp.	Pertussis	A macrolide	Ampicillin; TMP/SMX
Borrelia spp.	Relapsing fever, Lyme disease	Tetracycline (Pts >7 yrs)	Penicillin G; ceftriaxone; a macrolide
Brucella spp.	Brucellosis	Tetracycline (Pts >7 yrs); (+ gentamicin, if severe)	Chloramphenicol; TMP/SMX; rifampin
Burkholderia cepacia	(See *Pseudomonas cepacia*)		
Calymmatobacterium granulomatis	Granuloma inguinale	Tetracycline (Pts >7 yrs)	Chloramphenicol; an aminoglycoside
Campylobacter spp.	Diarrhea	A macrolide; imipenem	Tetracycline (Pts >7 yrs); an aminoglycoside
	Sepsis, meningitis	An aminoglycoside	According to *in vitro* tests
Capnocytophaga canimorsus	Sepsis following dog bite	Penicillin G	A macrolide; a cephalosporin
Capnocytophaga ochraceae	Sepsis, abscesses	Penicillin G	A macrolide; cefoxitin; metronidazole
Chlamydia pneumoniae (TWAR)	Pneumonia	Tetracycline (Pts >7 yrs)	A macrolide
Chlamydia psittaci	Psittacosis	Tetracycline (Pts >7 yrs)	Chloramphenicol

45

Organism	Clinical Illness	Drug of Choice	Alternatives
Chlamydia trachomatis	Lymphogranuloma venereum	Tetracycline (Pts >7 yrs)	A macrolide; erythromycin
	Urethritis, vaginitis	Tetracycline (Pts >7 yrs)	Erythromycin; sulfonamide; ampicillin
	Inclusion conjunctivitis of newborn	Erythromycin (oral)	Topical erythromycin, tetracycline or sulfonamide
	Pneumonia in infancy	A macrolide	Ampicillin; sulfonamide
	Trachoma	Topical + oral tetracycline (Pts >7 yrs)	Topical + oral sulfonamide
Chromobacterium violaceum	Sepsis, pneumonia, abscesses	Chloramphenicol	None
Citrobacter spp.	Meningitis, sepsis	An aminoglycoside	A cephalosporin; TMP/SMX
Clostridium spp.	Tetanus, gas gangrene, sepsis	Penicillin G (+ antitoxin for tetanus)	Tetracycline (Pts >7 yrs); clindamycin; metronidazole
Clostridium difficile	Antibiotic-associated colitis	Vancomycin (oral) or metronidazole (oral)	Bacitracin (oral)
Corynebacterium diphtheriae	Diphtheria	Penicillin G (+ antitoxin)	A macrolide
Corynebacterium, JK group	Sepsis	Vancomycin	According to *in vitro* tests
Corynebacterium minutissimum	Erythrasma	Topical miconazole or clindamycin	A macrolide

46

Organism	Infection	Drug of choice	Alternative
Ehrlichia canis (*chafeensis*)	Ehrlichiosis	Tetracycline (Pts >7 yrs)	Chloramphenicol
E'kenella corrodens	Abscesses, meningitis	Tetracycline (Pts >7 yrs)	Ampicillin; aminoglycoside; a macrolide
Enterobacter spp.	Sepsis, pneumonia, wound infection	Ceftriaxone; cefotaxime	An aminoglycoside; imipenem; TMP/SMX
	Urinary infection	TMP/SMX	An aminoglycoside; nitrofurantoin
Enterococcus spp.	Endocarditis, urinary infection	Ampicillin + an aminoglycoside	Vancomycin + an aminoglycoside
Erysipelothrix insidiosa	Sepsis, cellulitis, abscesses	Ampicillin (?) plus aminoglycoside	Tetracycline (Pts >7 yrs)
Escherichia coli	Urinary infection, not hospital acquired	A sulfonamide	Ampicillin; amoxicillin; a cephalosporin
	Sepsis, meningitis, pneumonia, hospital acquired urinary infection	An aminoglycoside; a cephalosporin	TMP/SMX; imipenem
Flavobacterium meningosepticum	Sepsis, meningitis	Vancomycin	An aminoglycoside; TMP/SMX
Francisella tularensis	Tularemia	Gentamicin or streptomycin	Tetracycline (Pts >7 yrs); chloramphenicol
Fusobacterium spp.	Sepsis, soft tissue infection	Penicillin G	Metronidazole; clindamycin
Gardnerella vaginalis	Genital infection	Metronidazole	Clindamycin

Organism	Clinical Illness	Drug of Choice	Alternatives
Haemophilus aphrophilus	Sepsis, endocarditis, abscesses	Tetracycline (Pts >7 yrs)	Ampicillin
Haemophilus ducreyi	Chancroid	Ceftriaxone	TMP/SMX; a macrolide
Haemophilus influenzae	Upper respiratory infections	Augmentin; erythromycin-sulfa; clarithromycin; oral cephalosporins; TMP/SMX	Amoxicillin (if beta-lactamase negative)
	Meningitis, arthritis, cellulitis, epiglottitis, pneumonia	Chloramphenicol; ceftriaxone; cefotaxime	Ampicillin (if beta-lactamase negative)
Helicobacter pylori	Gastritis, peptic ulcer	Amoxicillin + metronidazole + PeptoBismol	Other regimens incl ranitidine, omeprazole, clarithromycin
Herpes simplex virus	Keratoconjunctivitis	Trifluridine (topical)	Vidarabine (topical)
	Encephalitis, disseminated disease	Acyclovir	Vidarabine
Human immunodeficiency virus	AIDS, ARC	Zidovudine	Didanosine; zalcitabine
Influenza A virus	Influenza	Amantadine	(?) Ribavirin
Klebsiella spp.	Urinary tract infection	TMP/SMX	A cephalosporin; nitrofurantoin
	Sepsis, pneumonia, meningitis	Ceftriaxone; cefotaxime	An aminoglycoside; TMP/SMX; imipenem
Legionella spp.	Legionnaires' disease and related illnesses	A macrolide + rifampin	TMP/SMX; ciprofloxacin

Organism	Infection	Drug of choice	Alternative
		Penicillin G	Clindamycin; tetracycline (Pts >7 yrs)
Listeria monocytogenes	Sepsis, meningitis	Ampicillin (?) plus aminoglycoside	TMP/SMX
Moraxella catarrhalis	Otitis, sinusitis, bronchitis	Augmentin; a macrolide	TMP/SMX; a cephalosporin
Moraxella other spp.	Bone and joint infection; abscess	Penicillin G	Ampicillin; an aminoglycoside
Morganella morganii	Urinary infection, sepsis	An aminoglycoside	A cephalosporin
Mycobacterium tuberculosis	Tuberculosis	Isoniazid and rifampin (? + pyrazinamide)	An aminoglycoside; cycloserine; ethambutol; ethionamide
Mycobacteria, nontuberculous ("atypical")	Cervical adenitis	None (Surgery)	Rifampin; clarithromycin
	Other diseases	Rifampin; an aminoglycoside; clofazimine (multiple drug therapy)	Clarithromycin; azithromycin
Mycobacterium marinum (*M. balnei*)	Papules, pustules, cold abscesses (Swimmer's granuloma)	(?) TMP/SMX; rifampin	None (usually self-limited)
Mycobacterium leprae	Leprosy	Dapsone + rifampin + clofazimine	Clarithromycin
Mycoplasma hominis	Non-gonococcal urethritis	Clindamycin	Tetracycline (Pts >7 yrs)
Mycoplasma pneumoniae	Pneumonia	A macrolide	Tetracycline (Pts >7 yrs)
Neisseria gonorrhoeae beta-lactamase negative	Gonorrhea	Amoxicillin + probenecid;	Penicillin G

Organism	Clinical Illness	Drug of Choice	Alternatives
N. gonorrhoeae, beta-lactamase positive	Gonorrhea	Ceftriaxone; spectinomycin	TMP/SMX; other cephalosporins
Neisseria meningitidis	Sepsis, meningitis	Penicillin G	Ampicillin; chloramphenicol; a sulfonamide (if susceptible); a cephalosporin
Nocardia asteroides	Nocardiosis	A sulfonamide (? amikacin initially)	Amikacin; TMP/SMX; cycloserine; a macrolide
Pasteurella multocida	Sepsis, abscesses	Penicillin G	Tetracycline (Pts >7 yrs); ampicillin
Peptostreptococcus	Sepsis	Penicillin G	Clindamycin; vancomycin
Plesiomonas shigelloides	Diarrhea, meningitis	TMP/SMX	An aminoglycoside
Propionibacterium acnes	Sepsis, skin lesions	Penicillin G	Tetracycline; clindamycin; a macrolide; cephalosporin
Proteus mirabilis	Urinary infection, sepsis, meningitis	Ampicillin	An aminoglycoside; TMP/SMX; cephalosporin
Proteus, other spp.	Urinary infection, sepsis, meningitis	Cefotaxime; ceftriaxone	Imipenem; an aminoglycoside
Providencia spp.	Sepsis	Cefotaxime; ceftriaxone	TMP/SMX; imipenem; an aminoglycoside
Pseudomonas aeruginosa	Urinary infection	Anti-Pseudomonas beta-lactam	An aminoglycoside; imipenem
	Sepsis, pneumonia	Anti-Pseudomonas beta-lactam + an aminoglycoside	Imipenem; ciprofloxacin

Organism	Disease	Drug of Choice	Alternatives
Pseudomonas (Burkholderia) cepacia	Pneumonia, sepsis	TMP/SMX; ceftazidime	According to *in vitro* tests
Pseudomonas mallei	Glanders	Tetracycline (Pts >7 yrs) + streptomycin	Chloramphenicol; gentamicin
Pseudomonas pseudomallei	Melioidosis	Ceftazidime OR chloramphenicol + sulfa + aminoglycoside for sepsis	TMP/SMX or tetracycline (Pts >7 yrs) for chronic disease
Respiratory syncytial virus	Bronchiolitis, pneumonia	Ribavirin	None
Rhodococcus equi	Necrotizing pneumonia	Vancomycin	An aminoglycoside; a macrolide; chloramphenicol
Rickettsia	Rocky Mountain spotted fever, Q fever, typhus, rickettsialpox, ehrlichiosis	Tetracycline (Pts >7 years)	Chloramphenicol; ciprofloxacin
Rochalimaea henselae, R. quintana	Cat-scratch disease, bacillary angiomatosis, peliosis hepatis	A macrolide	TMP/SMX; tetracycline; gentamicin
Salmonella spp.	Focal infections, typhoid fever, sepsis	TMP/SMX; chloramphenicol; ceftriaxone	Ampicillin (if susceptible)
Serratia marcescens	Sepsis, pneumonia	Ceftriaxone; cefotaxime	TMP/SMX; an aminoglycoside; imipenem
Shigella spp.	Enteritis, urinary infection, vaginitis	TMP/SMX	Ampicillin; tetracycline (Pts >7 yrs); chloramphenicol
Spirillum minus	Rat bite fever (sodoku)	Penicillin G	Tetracycline (Pts >7 yrs); an aminoglycoside

Organism	Clinical Illness	Drug of Choice	Alternatives
Staphylococcus aureus	Skin infections	Cefadroxil; other oral cephalosporins	Cloxacillin; a macrolide; Augmentin
	Pneumonia, sepsis, osteomyelitis, etc.	Nafcillin	A cephalosporin; vancomycin; clindamycin; Timentin;
	Methicillin-resistant strains	Vancomycin (? + rifampin or aminoglycoside)	TMP/SMX; ciprofloxacin
Staphylococcus, coagulase negative	Sepsis, infected CNS shunts, urinary infection	Vancomycin	If susceptible: nafcillin (or related drug); (?) TMP/SMX
Staphylococcus spp., methicillin-resistant	Sepsis, focal infections	Vancomycin (?) + rifampin and/or gentamicin	TMP/SMX; ciprofloxacin
Streptobacillus moniliformis	Rat bite fever (Haverhill fever)	Penicillin G	Tetracycline (Pts >7 yrs); an aminoglycoside
Streptococcus, Groups A, B, C, and G, anaerobic	Pharyngitis, impetigo, adenitis	Penicillin V or benzathine penicillin	A macrolide; a cephalosporin; clindamycin
	Pneumonia, sepsis, meningitis	Penicillin G or ampicillin	A cephalosporin; vancomycin
Streptococcus, viridans group	Endocarditis	Penicillin G + gentamicin	Vancomycin; a cephalosporin
Streptococcus pneumoniae	Pneumonia, otitis	Penicillin V or G	A macrolide; a cephalosporin
	Meningitis, arthritis, sepsis	Penicillin G	Vancomycin (for penicillin-resistant strains); chloramphenicol, cephalosporin for

Organism	Disease	Drug of choice	Alternative
Treponema pallidum	Syphilis	Penicillin G	Tetracycline (Pts >7 yrs); ceftriaxone; a macrolide
Treponema pertenue	Yaws	Penicillin G	Tetracycline (Pts >7 yrs)
Ureaplasma urealyticum	Genitourinary infections	A macrolide	Tetracycline (Pts >7 yrs)
Varicella-zoster virus	Disseminated disease; zoster (shingles)	Acyclovir	Vidarabine
Vibrio cholerae	Cholera	Tetracycline (Pts >7 yrs)	TMP/SMX
Vibrio vulnificus	Sepsis	Tetracycline (Pts >7 yrs)	A cephalosporin
Xanthomonas maltophilia	Sepsis	An aminoglycoside + rifampin	TMP/SMX; ceftazidime
Yersinia enterocolitica	Enteritis, arthritis, sepsis	? Tetracycline (Pts >7 yrs); TMP/SMX	A macrolide; an aminoglycoside
Yersinia pestis	Plague	Streptomycin + chloramphenicol or tetracycline (Pts >7 yrs)	Other aminoglycoside
Yersinia pseudotuberculosis	Adenitis	? Tetracycline	? TMP/SMX

53

VIII. ANTIFUNGAL THERAPY

Infection	Therapy	Comments
SYSTEMIC INFECTIONS		
Aspergillosis	Amphotericin B initial dose 0.5 mg/kg IV in 3-4 hour infusion in 5% dextrose sol'n (no saline). Increase daily dosage by 0.25 mg/kg increments to maximum daily dosage of 1 mg/kg. Total dosage 30-35 mg/kg given over period of 4-6 weeks or longer. (For allergic bronchopulmonary aspergillosis see page 28)	Treat only for tissue invasion, not colonization; Monitor renal function, potassium and hemoglobin; Azotemia common; Rapidly advancing disease may require short-term use of doses to 1.5 mg/kg/day; Total dosage and duration of therapy individualized
Blastomycosis (North American)	Itraconazole 200-400 mg/day (adults), (?) 4 mg/kg/day (pediatric dosage not established) PO OR amphotericin B (as above) for severe disease	Treat only progressive or severe disease; Alternative: ketoconazole 6 mg/kg/day PO div q12-24 hr x 6 months
Candidiasis		
- Disseminated infection	Amphotericin B (as above) but daily dosage 0.5-0.75 mg/kg OR amphotericin B PLUS flucytosine 100-150 mg/kg/day PO div q6h	Hematologic toxicity and diarrhea with flucytosine
- Urinary infection	Fluconazole 3-6 mg/kg once daily OR flucytosine 50 mg/kg/day div q6h	Stopping antibiotic or removing Foley catheter sometimes leads to spontaneous cure in the normal host

54

Condition	Treatment	Alternative/Notes
- Oropharyngeal, esophageal	Clotrimazole 10 mg troche PO 5 x daily x 7 days OR fluconazole 3 mg/kg once daily	Amphotericin B for severe disease or febrile neutropenic pts
Chromomycosis	Flucytosine OR ketoconazole (as above)	
Coccidioidomycosis	Amphotericin B (as above) OR (for non-life threatening disease) 400 mg daily (adults) ketoconazole or itraconazole OR fluconazole 6 mg/kg once daily	Fluconazole or intrathecal amphotericin B for meningitis
Cryptococcosis	Amphotericin B 0.5-0.7 mg/kg IV daily OR flucytosine 100-150 mg/kg/day PO div q6h PLUS amphotericin B 0.3-0.5 mg/kg IV daily 6 weeks or longer	For HIV-positive, fluconazole 6 mg/kg daily, then 3 mg/kg daily maintenance
Histoplasmosis	Amphotericin B (as for aspergillosis) OR (for non-life threatening disease) itraconazole 200 mg b.i.d. PO (adults)	Ketoconazole (as above) as alternative
Mucormycosis (zygomycosis)	Amphotericin B (as for aspergillosis) x 6 wks or longer	Surgery, as necessary; Intrathecal amphotericin B may be needed for CNS infection
Paracoccidioidomycosis	Itraconazole 100 mg/day PO (adult OR amphotericin B (as for aspergillosis)	Ketoconazole (as above) as alternative; Sulfa drugs less effective but inexpensive
Phaeohyphomycosis	Amphotericin B (as for aspergillosis) x 3 wks or longer	Surgery, as necessary

Infection	Therapy	Comments
Pneumocystis carinii pneumonia	Trimethoprim-sulfamethoxazole 15-20 mg TMP-75-100 mg SMX/kg/day IV, PO div q6h **OR** pentamidine isethionate 4 mg base/kg/day IV daily x 10-14 days; Alternatives: trimethoprim and dapsone; primaquine and clindamycin; trimetrexate and folinic acid; atovaquone	Prophylaxis: 5 mg TMP-25 mg SMX/kg/day once daily PO **OR** 300 mg aerosolized pentamidine once monthly (adult dosage; dosage for children not established)
Pseudallescheria boydii and Scedosporium apiospermum infection	Miconazole 20-40 mg/kg/day IV div q8h x 3 weeks or longer	Ketoconazole or itraconazole may be effective
Sporotrichosis	Itraconazole 100-20 mg/day PO (adult dosage); amphotericin B (as for aspergillosis) for severe disease	Alternative: Sat. sol'n of potassium iodide 1-2 drops per year of age 3 x daily PO (maximum 30 drops t.i.d.) until lymphocutaneous lesions resolved (give with fruit juice or milk)

LOCALIZED MUCOCUTANEOUS INFECTIONS

Dermatophytoses

- Scalp (including kerion)	Griseofulvin microcrystalline 10-15 mg/kg once daily x 1-2 mos or longer (Taken with milk or fatty foods to augment absorption) **OR** ketoconazole 6 mg/kg/day div q12-24h	Topical antifungal agent does not help heal acute stage but may prevent recurrence from endothrix spores; Selsun shampoo twice weekly may be useful adjunct
- Glabrous skin, hands or feet	Topical econazole, miconazole, clotrimazole, ketoconazole or ciclopirox applied 2x daily x 7-10 days (longer for palmar/plantar infections)	

	Therapy	Comments
- Tinea versicolor	Selenium sulfide (Selsun) OR topical clotrimazole (or related drug) applied twice daily x 7-10 days	Recurrence common; Ketoconazole useful for extensive lesions
Candidiasis		
- Benign mucocutaneous	Topical ketoconazole, econazole, nystatin, clotrimazole or miconazole 3-4 x daily x 7-10 days	0.5% aqueous gentian violet for refractory cases
- Oral thrush	Nystatin suspension in mouth 3-4 x daily after feedings x 7-10 days	
- Chronic mucocutaneous	Ketoconazole 6 mg/kg/day PO div q12-24h OR fluconazole 3 mg/kg daily PO until lesions clear	Occurs in hosts with variety of immune defects
- Vulvovaginal	Vaginal cream with butoconazole, clotrimazole, miconazole, terconazole or tioconazole; OR vaginal tablets/ suppositories of clotrimazole, miconazole, terconazole; all at bedtime x 3-7 days	

IX. ANTIPARASITIC THERAPY

Note: Familiarize yourself with the toxic potentials of these drugs and monitor the patient accordingly. For some of the parasitic diseases, drugs available only from the Centers for Disease Control are the preferred therapy. These drugs are indicated by "(CDC)". Consultation for diagnostic tests and detailed information about experimental drugs are available around the clock from the CDC and they will send drugs to you. The telephone number during the day is 404-639-3670. Nights and weekends call 404-639-2888 and ask the duty officer for the Parasitic Disease Drug Service doctor on call.

Disease/Organism	Treatment
AMEBIASIS *Entamoeba histolytica*	
- Asymptomatic carrier	Iodoquinol (formerly diiodohydroxyquin) 40 mg/kg/day (max 2 g) PO div q8h x 20 days; OR diloxanide furoate (CDC) 20 mg/kg/day PO div q8h x 10 days OR paromomycin 30 mg/kg/day PO div q8h x 7-10 days
- Mild to moderate colitis	Metronidazole 35-50 mg/kg/day PO div q8h x 10 days; OR paromomycin 30 mg/kg/day PO div q8h x 7-10 days; FOLLOWED BY iodoquinol as above, x 20 days
- Severe colitis	Metronidazole 35-50 mg/kg/day PO, IV div q8h x 10 days OR dehydroemetine (CDC) 1.0-1.5 mg/kg/day (max 90 mg) IM div q12h x 5 days EITHER DRUG FOLLOWED BY iodoquinol or paromomycin, as above
- Liver abscess and other extra- intestinal disease	Metronidazole, as above, x 10 days FOLLOWED BY iodoquinol, as above, x 20 days; OR dehydroemetine (CDC), as above, FOLLOWED BY chloroquine 10 mg base/kg/day (max 300 mg) PO x 14-21 days PLUS iodoquinol, or paromomycin, as above
AMEBIC MENINGOENCEPHALITIS *Naegleria* spp., *Acanthamoeba* spp., *Hartmannella* spp.	Amphotericin B 1 mg/kg/day IV x uncertain duration, (?) PLUS miconazole and rifampin for *Naegleria*; Intrathecal miconazole (10 mg) daily may be helpful; *Acanthamoeba* susceptible *in vitro* to ketoconazole, flucytosine, pentamidine

58

ANGIOSTRONGYLIASIS
Angiostrongylus spp.

Thiabendazole 50-75 mg/kg/day PO div q8h for *A. costaricensis*
x 3 days OR mebendazole 100 mg PO b.i.d. x 5 days for *A. cantonensis*

ANISAKIASIS
Anasakis spp.

Removal by fibroendoscopy or surgery

ASCARIASIS
Ascaris lumbricoides

Pyrantel pamoate 11 mg/kg PO (max 1 g) x 1 dose OR mebendazole 100 mg b.i.d.
x 3

BABESIOSIS
Babesia spp.

Clindamycin (30 mg/kg/day PO div q8h) PLUS quinine (25 mg/kg/day PO div q6h) x 7 days effective in limited experience; Exchange blood transfusion reported helpful; Pentamidine, TMP/SMX and azithromycin may be effective

BALANTIDIASIS
Balantidium coli

Metronidazole 35-50 mg/kg/day PO div q8h x 5 days OR tetracycline (Pts >7 yrs) 40 mg/kg/day PO div q6h x 10 days OR iodoquinol 40 mg/kg/day PO div q8h x 20 days

BLASTOCYSTIASIS
Blastocystis hominis

Metronidazole 35-50 mg/kg/day PO div q8h x 10 days OR iodoquinol 40 mg/kg/day (max 2 g) PO div q8h x 20 days (Based on anecdotal reports)

CAPILLARIASIS
Capillaria philippinensis

Mebendazole 200 mg PO b.i.d. x 20 days OR thiabendazole 25 mg/kg/day PO div q12h x 30 days

CHAGA'S DISEASE
Trypanosoma cruzi

See TRYPANOSOMIASIS

Clonorchis sinensis

(See FLUKES)

CRYPTOSPORIDIOSIS
Cryptosporidium parvum

No proved effective therapy; Spiramycin, paromomycin or azithromycin may be effective

59

Disease/Organism	Treatment
CUTANEOUS LARVA MIGRANS or CREEPING ERUPTION (Cutaneous hookworm)	Thiabendazole suspension topically b.i.d. x 2-5 days; OR thiabendazole 50 mg/kg/day PO div q12h x 3 days; Note: ethylene chloride spray and carbon dioxide snow are effective but painful and sometimes damage tissue
CYCLOSPORIASIS *Cyclospora* sp. (Cyanobacterium-like agent)	Trimethoprim-sulfamethoxazole (5 mg TMP-25 mg SMX/kg/day) PO div q12h x 3 days may be effective
CYSTICERCOSIS *Cysticercus cellulosae*	Praziquantel 50 mg/kg/day PO div q8h x 14 days; For CNS cysticercosis give steroids before first dose of praziquantel; (Praziquantel therapy is controversial); Albendazole may be effective
DIENTAMOEBIASIS *Dientamoeba fragilis*	Iodoquinol 40 mg/kg/day (max 2g) PO div q8h x 20 days; OR tetracycline (Pts >7 yrs) 40 mg/kg/day PO div q6h x 7-10 days
Diphyllobothrium latum	See TAPEWORMS
DIROFILARIASIS *Dirofilaria immitis*	Surgical excision of subcutaneous or pulmonary nodules; Praziquantel possibly effective
DRACUNCULOSIS *Dracunculus medinensis* (Guinea worm)	Metronidazole 25 mg/kg/day PO div q8h x 10 days; OR thiabendazole 50-75 mg/kg PO div q12h x 3 days; IN ADDITION remove worm by winding out a few cm each day
ECHINOCOCCOSIS *Echinococcus granulosus*	Surgical treatment when indicated; Albendazole (CDC) 15 mg/kg/day PO div q12h x 28 days
Entamoeba histolytica	See AMEBIASIS
Enterobius vermicularis	See PINWORMS
Fasciola hepatica	See FLUKES

60

FILARIASIS

- River blindness
  Onchocerca volvulus

Ivermectin (CDC) 150 mcg/kg (0.15 mg/kg) PO as single dose; Repeat q6-12mos; Antihistamines or corticosteroids for allergic reactions

- Other forms (Loa loa, tropical eosinophilia)
  Wuchereria bancrofti, Brugia malayi

Diethylcarbamazine 1 mg/kg on Day 1, 1 mg/kg t.i.d. on Day 2, 2 mg/kg t.i.d. on Day 3; then 6 mg/kg/day (9 mg/kg/day for loa loa) PO div q8h x 18 days; Antihistamines or corticosteroids for allergic reactions; surgical excision of subcutaneous nodules, preferably before drug therapy; Ivermectin (CDC) may be effective

FLUKES

- Sheep liver fluke (*Fasciola hepatica*)
- Lung fluke (*Paragonimus westermani*)
- Chinese liver fluke (*Clonorchis sinensis*) and others (*Fasciolopsis, Heterophyes, Metagonimus, Opisthorchis*)

Praziquantel 75 mg/kg PO div q8h x 1 day (x 2 days for *P. westermani*) is drug of choice for all fluke infections except *F. hepatica* for which bithionol (CDC) is given (30-50 mg/kg PO q.i.d. x 10-15 doses)

GIARDIASIS
Giardia lamblia

Furazolidone 6-8 mg/kg/day PO div q6h x 7-10 days OR quinacrine 6 mg/kg/day (max 300 mg/d) PO div q8h x 5 days; OR metronidazole 15 mg/kg/day PO div q8h x 5 days; (All can have Antabuse-like effect)

GNATHOSTOMIASIS
Gnathostoma spinigerum

Surgical removal OR mebendazole 200 mg PO q3h x 6 days

HOOKWORM
Necator americanus, Ancylostoma duodenale

Mebendazole 100 mg PO b.i.d. x 3 days; OR pyrantel pamoate 11 mg/kg (max 1 g/d) PO daily x 3 days

Hymenolepis nana

See TAPEWORMS

ISOSPORIASIS
Isospora belli

Trimethoprim-sulfamethoxazole 10 mg TMP-50 mg SMX/kg/day div q6h x 10 days; Then, 5 mg TMP-25 mg SMX/kg/day div q12h x 3 wks

61

Disease/Organism	Treatment
LEISHMANIASIS, including kala azar *Leishmania braziliensis,* *L. donovani, L. tropica, L. mexicana*	Stibogluconate sodium (CDC) 20 mg/kg/day IM or IV, daily x 20 days (10 mg/kg/day x 10 days for *L. tropica*); ALTERNATIVES, for L. *donovani*, pentamidine isethionate 4 mg/kg/day IM daily for 14 days; OR, for *L. mexicana*, amphotericin B 1 mg/kg/day IV x 4-8 wks; ketaconazole was effective for *L. mexicana* in one report; (Concomitant treatment with interferon gamma has been used for refractory cases of visceral disease)
LICE *Pediculus capitis or humanus,* *Phthirus pubis*	Permethrin 1% (Nix Creme Rinse) OR pyrethins (RID, A-200 Pyrinate liquid or shampoo, R & C Shampoo) OR lindane (Kwell) applied topically once (follow manufacturer's instructions for use); Repeat in 1 wk; For eyelash infestation, use petrolatum; Launder bedding and clothing
MALARIA	CDC Malaria Hotline (24 hrs a day) 404/332-4555
Prophylaxis - For areas without chloroquine-resistant *P. falciparum*	Chloroquine or amodiaquine 5 mg base/kg (max 300 mg) PO once weekly, beginning 1 week before arrival in malarial zone and continuing for 4 weeks after last exposure (drugs available in liquid form outside the USA); PLUS (optional) beginning with final 2 weeks of chloroquine Rx, primaquine 0.3 mg base/kg PO daily x 14 days after departure from endemic area for individuals heavily exposed to mosquitoes
- For areas where chloroquine-resistant *P. falciparum* exists	Chloroquine (as above); Have pyrimethamine-sulfadoxine (Fansidar) available to take if febrile illness develops; OR mefloquine for children >45 kg 250 mg once weekly starting 1 week before travel and for 4 weeks after leaving area; for children 15-19 kg, 1/4 tab; 20-30 kg, 1/2 tab; 31-45 kg, 3/4 tab; OR doxycycline (Pt > 7 yr) 2 mg/kg (max 100 mg) daily
Treatment of disease - *Plasmodium vivax, P. ovale* *P. malariae,* chloroquine-susceptible *P. falciparum*	Chloroquine 10 mg base/kg (max 600 mg) PO stat, then 5 mg base/kg at 6 hrs, 24 hrs and 48 hrs after initial dose; For parenteral therapy, quinidine 10 mg/kg (max 600 mg) IV (1 hr infusion) followed by continuous infusion of 0.02 mg/kg/min until oral therapy can be given (3 days maximum); Prevention of

62

- _P. falciparum_
chloroquine-resistant

Quinine 25 mg/kg/day (max 2 g/day) PO div q8h x 3 days **AND** Fansidar (pyrimethamine-sulfadoxine): <1 yr, 1/4 tab; 1-3 yrs, 1/2 tab; 4-8 yrs, 1 tab; 9-14 yrs, 2 tab; >14 yrs, 3 tab as a single dose on last day of quinine; NOTE: Several alternative regimens have been reported for Fansidar-resistant infections: Check with the CDC; For parenteral therapy, quinidine, as above; <u>NOTE</u>: Corticosteroids are contraindicated in cerebral malaria; Iron chelation therapy may be beneficial in cerebral malaria

Paragonimus westermani

See FLUKES

PINWORMS
Enterobius vermicularis

Pyrantel pamoate 11 mg/kg (max 1 g) PO x 1 dose <u>OR</u> mebendazole 100 mg PO x 1 dose; repeat treatment in 2 weeks

PNEUMOCYSTIS PNEUMONIA
Pneumocystis carinii

See page 56

SCABIES
Sarcoptes scabei

Permethrin 5% cream applied to entire body (incl scalp in infants), left on for 8-14 hr before bathing; <u>OR</u> lindane (Kwell) lotion applied to all of body below neck, leave on overnight, bathe in a.m.; Launder bedding and clothing; Topical corticosteroid <u>after</u> treatment for severe, persistent itching

SCHISTOSOMIASIS
Schistosoma hematobium, japonicum, mansoni, mekongi

Praziquantel 40-60 mg/kg/day PO in 2-3 doses taken in 1 day

STRONGYLOIDIASIS
Strongyloides stercoralis

Thiabendazole 50 mg/kg/day (max 3 g/d) PO div q12h x 2 days (5 days or longer for disseminated disease); Invermectin (CDC) may be effective

TAPEWORMS

- _Cysticercus cellulosae_

See CYSTICERCOSIS

Disease/Organism	Treatment
- *Echinococcus granulosus*	See ECHINOCOCCOSIS
- *Taenia saginata, T. solium, Hymenolepis nana, Diphyllobothrium latum, Dipylidium carinum*	Praziquantel 5-10 mg/kg x 1 dose (25 mg/kg for *H. nana*) OR niclosamide tablet approx 40 mg/kg PO chewed thoroughly x 1 dose (for *H. nana* treat for 6 days)
TOXOPLASMOSIS *Toxoplasma gondii*	Pyrimethamine 2 mg/kg/day PO q12h x 3 days, then 1 mg/kg/day (max 25 mg every other day) PO (Supplemental folinic acid) AND trisulfapyrimidines or sulfadiazine 120 mg/kg/day PO div q6h; OR spiramycin (CDC) 50-100 mg/kg/day PO div q6h; Treatment continued for 4 wks after resolution of illness (See page 8 for congenital toxoplasmosis); Corticosteroids given for ocular infection
TRICHINOSIS *Trichinella spiralis*	Anti-inflammatory drugs; steroids for CNS or severe symptoms; Mebendazole 200-400 mg t.i.d. x 3 days, then 400-500 mg t.i.d. x 10 d
TRICHOMONIASIS *Trichomonas vaginalis*	Metronidazole 40 mg/kg (max 2 g) PO x 1 dose; OR metronidazole 15 mg/kg/day (max 1 g/day) PO div q8h x 7 days; Treat sex partners
TRICHOSTRONGYLIASIS *Trichostrongylus orientalis*	Pyrantel pamoate 11 mg/kg (max 1 g) PO x 1 dose OR mebendazole 100 mg bid x 3 days
Trichuris trichiura	See WHIPWORM
TRYPANOSOMIASIS *Trypanosoma cruzi*	
- **CHAGA'S DISEASE**	Nifurtimox (CDC) or benznidazole (CDC); Obtain dosage recommendations from CDC
- **SLEEPING SICKNESS** *T. brucei gambiense; T. brucei rhodesiense*	Acute stage: suramin (CDC) 20 mg/kg IV on days 1, 3, 7, 14 and 21 OR pentamidine isethionate 4 mg/kg/day IV x 10 days Late disease with CNS involvement: melarsoprol (CDC) initial dose 0.36

VISCERAL LARVA MIGRANS
Toxocara canis; T. cati

Thiabendazole 50 mg/kg/day PO div q12h x 5 days or longer; Corticosteroids for severe symptoms and for eye infection; <u>OR</u> diethylcarbamazine 6 mg/kg/day div q8h x 7-10 days

WHIPWORM (TRICHURIASIS)
Trichuris trichiura

Mebendazole 100 mg PO b.i.d. x 3 days

Wuchereria bancrofti

See FILARIASIS

PARASITES OF MINOR OR NO MEDICAL IMPORTANCE

These organisms are commensal or cause minor symptoms that usually do not require therapy.

NEMATODES

Capillaria hepatica, Dioctophyma renale, Dipetalonema perstans, Dipetolonema streptocerca, Mansonella ozzardi, Syngamus larnygeus, Termides deminutus

FLAGELLATE PROTOZOA

Chilomastix mesnili, Enteromonas hominis, Retortamonas intestindlis, Trichomonas hominis, Trichomonas tenax

AMEBAE

Endolimax nana, Entamoeba coli, Entamoeba gingivalis, Entamoeba hartmanni, Entamoeba polecki, Iodamoeba buetschlii

X. ALPHABETICAL LISTING OF ANTIBIOTICS WITH DOSAGE FORMS AND USUAL DOSAGES

NOTES:
1. When a range of dosage is given, the higher dosages are generally indicated for serious illnesses.
2. In some cases the dosages indicated differ from the manufacturers' recommendations in the package inserts.
3. IV preparations available in ready-to-use "piggy-back" bottles are not included in the tabulated dosage forms.

Generic and Trade® Names	Dosage Form	Route	Dosage	Interval
Acyclovir Zovirax®	500 mg vial 200 mg/5 ml susp	IV PO	25-50 mg/kg/day 80 mg/kg/day	q8h q6h
	200 mg cap; 400, 800 mg tab	PO	1 cap 5 times daily; 1 tab 4 times daily	
Amantadine HCl Symmetrel®	100 mg cap 50 mg/5 ml syrup	PO	5-8 mg/kg/day (max. 200 mg/day)	q12h
Amikacin sulfate Amikin®	0.1, 0.5, 1 g vials	IM, IV	15-22.5 mg/kg/day	q8h
Amoxicillin trihydrate Amoxil® Polymox®, Trimox®, Wymox®, generic	250, 500 mg cap 125, 250 mg/5 ml susp	PO	40 mg/kg/day	q8h
Amoxicillin and clavulanate potassium Augmentin®	"Augmentin 125" (125 mg amox + 31.25 mg clav)/5 ml susp; also chewable tab "Augmentin 250" (250 mg amox + 62.5 mg clav)/5 ml susp; also chewable tab "Augmentin 250" (250 mg amox + 125 mg clav) tab; "Augmentin 500" (500 mg	PO	40 mg amox component/ kg/day	q8h

Drug	Formulation	Route	Dosage	Frequency
Amphotericin B Fungizone®	50 mg vial	IV	0.25-1 mg/kg/day	q1-2 days
Ampicillin and Ampicillin trihydrate Omnipen®, Polycillin®, Principen®, generic	250, 500 mg cap 125 mg chewable tab 125, 250, 500 mg/5 ml susp 100 mg/ml drops	PO	50 mg/kg/day	q6h
Ampicillin, sodium Omnipen®, Polycillin®, generic	0.125, 0.25, 0.5, 1, 2, 4 g vials	IM, IV	100-200 mg/kg/day (meningitis 200-400)	q6h
Ampicillin/Sulbactam Unasyn®	1 g amp/0.5 g sul, 2 g amp/1 g sul	IV	As per ampicillin; not approved for children	q6h
Atovaquone Meprone®	250 mg tab	PO	750 mg/day (adult dosage)	q8h
Azithromycin Zithromax®	250 cap	PO	500 mg 1st day; then 250 mg (Pt > 15 yrs)	q24h
Aztreonam Azactam®	0.5, 1, 2 g vials	IM, IV	90-120 mg/kg/day	q6-8h
Bacampicillin HCl Spectrobid®	400 mg tab (equiv to 280 mg ampicillin) 125 mg/5 ml susp	PO	25-50 mg/kg/day	q12h
Bactracin	10,000, 50,000 unit vials	IM	800-1200 u/kg/day (not recommended)	q8h
Carbenicillin indanyl sodium Geocillin®	382 mg tab	PO	30-50 mg/kg/day	q6h

Generic and Trade® Names	Dosage Form	Route	Dosage	Interval
Cefaclor Ceclor®	125, 187, 250, 375 mg/5 ml susp 250, 500 mg cap	PO	40 mg/kg/day	q8-12h
Cefadroxil monohydrate Duricef®, Ultracef®, generic	500 mg cap, 1 g tab 125, 250, 500 mg/5 ml susp	PO	30 mg/kg/day	q12h
Cefamandole nafate Mandol®	0.5, 1, 2 g vials	IV, IM	100-150 mg/kg/day	q4-6h
Cefazolin sodium Ancef®, Kefzol®, Zolicef®, generic	0.25, 0.5, 1 g vials	IM, IV	50-100 mg/kg/day	q8h
Cefixime Suprax®	200, 400 mg tab 100 mg/5 ml susp	PO	8 mg/kg/day	q12-24h
Cefmetazole sodium Zefazone®	1, 2 g vials	IV	No established dosage for children	q8-12h
Cefonicid sodium Monocid®	0.5, 1 g vials	IV, IM	(?) 20-40 mg/kg/day (not approved for children)	q24h
Cefoperazone Cefobid®	1, 2 g vials	IV, IM	100-150 mg/kg/day (not approved for children)	q8-12h
Cefotaxime sodium Claforan®	0.5, 1, 2 g vials	IV, IM	100-150 mg/kg/day (meningitis 200)	q6-8h
Cefotetan Cefotan®	1, 2 g vials	IV, IM	(?) 40-80 mg/kg/day (not approved for children)	q12h

68

Cefpodoxime proxetil Vantin®	100,200 mg tab 50, 100 mg/5 ml susp	PO	10 mg/kg/day (max 400 mg)	q12h
Cefprozil Cefzil®	250, 500 mg tab 125, 250 mg/5 ml susp	PO	30 mg/kg/day	q12h
Ceftazidime Fortaz®, Pentacef®, Tazicef®, Tazidime®	0.5, 1, 2 g vials	IV, IM	100-150 mg/kg/day (meningitis 150)	q8h
Ceftibuten Cedax®	400 mg cap 90 mg/5 ml susp	PO	9 mg/kg/day	q24h
Ceftizoxime sodium Cefizox®	1, 2 g vials	IV, IM	150-200 mg/kg/day	q6-8h
Ceftriaxone Rocephin®	0.25, 0.5, 1, 5, 10 g vials	IM, IV	50-100 mg/kg/day (meningitis 100)	q12-24h q12h
Cefuroxime Kefurox®, Zinacef®	0.75, 1.5 g vials	IV, IM	100-150 mg/kg/day (meningitis 240)	q8h q6h
Cefuroxime axetil Ceftin®	125, 250, 500 mg tab	PO	30 mg/kg/day (40 for otitis)	q12h
Cephalexin monohydrate Keflex®, Keftab®, generic	250, 500 mg tab 0.25, 0.5, 1 g cap 100 mg/ml drops 125, 250 mg/5 ml susp	PO	25-50 mg/kg/day	q6h
Cephalothin, sodium	1, 2, 4 g vials	IM, IV	75-125 mg/kg/day	q4-6h
Cephapirin, sodium Cefadyl®	1, 2, 4 g vials	IM, IV	40-80 mg/kg/day	q6h

69

Generic and Trade® Names	Dosage Form	Route	Dosage	Interval
Cephradine Velosef®, generic	250, 500 mg cap 125, 250 mg/5 ml susp	PO	25-50 mg/kg/day	q6h
Chloramphenicol Chloramphenicol palmitate Chloromycetin®, generic	250 mg cap 150 mg/5 ml susp	PO	50-75 mg/kg/day (meningitis 75-100)	q6h
Chloramphenicol sodium succinate Chloromycetin®	1 g vial	IV		
Chloroquine HCl Aralen HCl®	250 mg amp (equiv to 200 mg base)	IM	5 mg base/kg	1 or 2 doses
Chloroquine PO$_4$ Aralen PO$_4$®, generic	500 mg tab (equiv to 300 mg base)	PO	10 mg base/kg/day	q24h
Chloroquine, hydroxy Plaquenil®	200 mg tab (equiv to 155 mg base)			
Ciprofloxacin Cipro®	250, 500, 750 mg tab	PO	20-30 mg/kg/day	q12h (not approved for < 18 yrs)
	200, 400 mg vial	IV	(?) 10-15 mg/kg/day	
Clarithromycin Biaxin®	250, 500 mg tab 125, 250 mg/5 ml susp	PO	15 mg/kg/day	q12h
Clindamycin HCl hydrate Clindamycin palmitate HCl	75, 150, 300 mg cap 75 mg/5 ml sol'n	PO	20-30 mg/kg/day	q6h
Clindamycin phosphate Cleocin®, generic	0.15, 0.3, 0.6 g amp	IM, IV	25-40 mg/kg/day	q6-8h

Drug	Formulation	Route	(adult dosage)	Frequency
Lamprene®				
Cloxacillin, sodium Cloxapen®, Tegopen®, generic	250, 500 mg cap 125 mg/5 ml sol'n	PO	50-100 mg/kg/day	q6h
Colistimethate, sodium Coly-Mycin M®	150 mg vial	IM, IV	5-7 mg/kg/day	q8h
Cycloserine Seromycin®	250 mg cap	PO	(?) 7-10 mg/kg/day (No recommended dosage for children)	q12h
Dapsone	25, 100 mg scored tab	PO	1 mg/kg/day	q24h
Demeclocycline HCl Declomycin®	150 mg cap 150, 300 mg tab	PO	8-12 mg/kg/day	q6-12h
Dicloxacillin monohydrate, sodium Dycill®, Dynapen®, Pathocil®, generic	125, 250, 500 mg cap 62.5 mg/5 ml susp	PO	12-25 mg/kg/day	q6h
Didanosine Videx®	250, 1000 g vials 25, 50, 100, 150 mg tab Powder for oral solution	IV PO	(?) 180 mg/m²/day According to BSA (see package insert)	q8h
Diiodohydroxyquin (See Iodoquinol)				
Doxycycline hyclate Doryx®, Vibramycin®, Vibra-Tabs®, generic	50, 100 mg cap	PO	2-4 mg/kg/day (Pts > 7 yrs)	q12h on 1st day; then 1/2 dose q24h
Doxycycline calcium Vibramycin®	50 mg/5 ml syrup			
Doxycycline monohydrate Vibramycin®	25 mg/5 ml susp			

71

Generic and Trade® Names	Dosage Form	Route	Dosage	Interval
Doxycycline hyclate Vibramycin®	100 mg vials	IV	2-4 mg/kg/day (Pts >7 yrs)	q24h as 2 hr infusion
Enoxacin Penetrex®	200, 400 mg tab	PO	400-800 mg/day (adult dosage)	q12h
Erythromycin E-Mycin®, ERYC®, Ery-Tab®, Erythromycin Base Filmtab®, Ilotycin®, PCE Dispertab®, generic	125 mg pellets in cap 250 mg tab, cap 333 mg tab 2% topical sol'n for acne 0.5% ophthalmic ung	PO Topical Topical	40 mg/kg/day	q6h
Erythromycin estolate Ilosone®, generic	100 mg/ml drops 500 mg tab 125, 250 mg cap 125, 250 mg chewable tab 125, 250 mg/5 ml susp	PO	30-40 mg/kg/day	q8-12h
Erythromycin ethylsuccinate E.E.S.®, EryPed®, Wyamycin E®	400 mg tab 200 mg chewable tab 200, 400 mg/5 ml susp 100 mg/2.5 ml drops	PO	40 mg/kg/day	q8h
Erythromycin ethylsuccinate and sulfisoxazole acetyl Pediazole®, Eryzole®	200 mg erythromycin and 600 mg sulfisoxazole/5 ml susp	PO	40 mg/kg/day of erythromycin component	q6-8h
Erythromycin gluceptate Ilotycin Gluceptate®	0.25, 0.5, 1 g amp	IV	20-50 mg/kg/day	contin- uous infusion;

			(1-2 hr infusion)
Erythromycin stearate Erythrocin Stearate®, Wyamycin S®, generic	250, 500 mg tab	PO	20-40 mg/kg/day	q6h
Ethambutol hydrochloride Myambutol®	100, 400 mg tab	PO	15 mg/kg/day	q24h
Ethionamide Trecator-SC®	250 mg tab	PO	(?) 10-20 mg/kg/day (No established dosage for children)	q12h
Fluconazole Diflucan®	50, 100, 200 mg tab 200, 400 mg vial	PO IV	(?) 3-6 mg/kg/day (No established dosage for children)	q24h
Flucytosine Ancobon®	250, 500 mg cap	PO	50-150 mg/kg/day	q6h
Foscarnet Foscavir®	6, 12 g vials	IV	Initial: 180 mg/kg/day Maintenance: 90 mg/kg/day	q8h q24h
Furazolidone Furoxone®	100 mg tab 50 mg/15 ml susp (contains kaolin and pectin)	PO	5-8 mg/kg/day	q6h
Ganciclovir Cytovene®	500 mg vial	IV	Induction; 10 mg/kg/day	q12h (1-2 hr infusion)
			Maintenance: 5 mg/kg/day (No established dosage for children)	q24h

Generic and Trade® Names	Dosage Form	Route	Dosage	Interval
Gentamicin sulfate Garamycin®, generic	20, 80 mg vials	IM, IV	3-7.5 mg/kg/day (cystic fibrosis 7-10)	q8h
Garamycin Intrathecal®	4 mg vial (intrathecal)	Intra-thecal	1-2 mg/day	q24h
Griseofulvin Fulvicin-P/G®, Fulvicin-U/F® Grifulvin V®, Grisactin®, Gris-PEG®	microsize: 125, 250, 500 mg tab, cap 125 mg/5 ml susp ultramicrosize: 125, 250 mg tab	PO	15 mg/kg/day	q24h
Imipenem-Cilastatin Primaxin®	250/250, 500/500 mg vials	IM, IV	40-60 mg/kg/day (not approved for children)	q6h
Idoquinol Yodoxin®	650 mg tab	PO	40 mg/kg/day	q8h
Isoniazid INH®, Laniazid®, generic	100, 300 mg scored lab 1 g vial 50 mg/5 ml syrup	PO, IM	10-20 mg/kg/day (max. 300 mg)	q12-24h
Isoniazid and pyridoxine	10 mg/0.5 mg/ml syrup	PO	(See isoniazid)	
Itraconazole Sporanox®	100 mg cap	PO	200-400 mg/day (adult dosage)	q24h
Kanamycin sulfate Kantrex®, generic	75 mg, 0.5, 1 g vials	IM, IV	15-30 mg/kg/day	q8h
	500 mg cap	PO	150-250 mg/kg/day (for suppression of bowel flora)	q1-6h

74

Nizoral®	250, 500 mg cap	PO	30-60 mg/kg/day	q8h
Lincomycin hydrochloride Lincocin®	0.6, 3 g vials	IM, IV	10-20 mg/kg/day	q8-12h
Lomefloxacin HCl Maxaquin®	400 mg tab	PO	400 mg/day (adult dosage)	q24h
Loracarbef Lorabid®	200 mg cap 100, 200 mg/5 ml susp	PO	30 (otitis)-15 (other indications) mg/kg/day	q12h
Mebendazole Vermox®	100 mg chewable tab	PO	See Section IX	
Mefloquine HCl Lariam®	250 mg tab	PO	See Section IX	
Methenamine hippurate Hiprex®, Urex®	1 g tab	PO	25-50 mg/kg/day	q12h
Methenamine mandelate Mandelamine®, Thiacide®, Uroquid®, generic	0.35, 0.5, 1 g tab 250, 500 mg/5 ml susp 0.5, 1 g granules	PO	50-75 mg/kg/day	q6h
Methicillin, sodium Staphcillin®	1, 4, 6 g vials	IM, IV	150-200 mg/kg/day	q6h
Metronidazole Flagyl®, Metric 21®, Protostat®, generic	250, 500 mg tab	PO	15-35 mg/kg/day	q8h
	500 mg vial	IV	30 mg/kg/day	q6h
Mezlocillin sodium Mezlin®	1, 2, 3, 4 g vials	IV	200-300 mg/kg/day	q4-6h

Generic and Trade® Names	Dosage Form	Route	Dosage	Interval
Miconazole Monistat®	200 mg amp	IV	20-40 mg/kg/day	q8h
Minocycline HCl Minocin®, generic	50, 100 mg pellet-filled cap 50 mg/5 ml susp	PO	4 mg/kg/day	q12h
	100 mg vial	IV	4 mg/kg/day	q12h
Mupirocin Bactroban®	15 g tube	Topical	Apply to infected skin	q8h
Nafcillin monohydrate, sodium Nafcil®, Unipen®, generic	250 mg cap, 500 mg tab 250 mg/5 ml sol'n	PO	50-100 mg/kg/day	q6h
Nalidixic acid NegGram®	0.5, 1, 2 g vials	IM, IV	150 mg/kg/day	q6h
	0.25, 0.5, 1 g tab 250 mg/5 ml susp	PO	55 mg/kg/day	q6h
Neomycin sulfate	500 mg tab 125 mg/5 ml sol'n	PO	50-100 mg/kg/day	q6-8h
Netilmicin Netromycin®	150 mg vials	IV, IM	3-7.5 mg/kg/day	q8h
Niclosamide Niclocide®	500 mg scored tab	PO	40 mg/kg/day	q24h
Nitrofurantoin Furadantin®	50, 100 mg scored tab 25 mg/5 ml susp	PO	5-7 mg/kg/day	q6h
Nitrofurantoin macrocrystals	25, 50, 100 mg cap	PO	5-7 mg/kg/day	q6h

76

Drug	Formulation	Route	Dosage	Frequency
Noroxin®			(adult dosage)	
Nystatin Mycostatin®, generic	100,000 u/ml susp 500,000 u tab	PO (not swallowed)	Infants 2 ml/dose; children 4-6 ml or 1 tab/dose	q6h
Ofloxacin Floxin®	200, 300, 400 mg tab 400 mg vial	PO	400-800 mg/day (adult dosage)	q12h
Oxacillin, sodium Bactocill®, Prostaphlin®, generic	250, 500 mg cap 250 mg/5 ml sol'n	PO	50-100 mg/kg/day	q6h
	0.25, 0.5, 1, 2, 4 g vials	IM, IV	150-200 mg/kg/day	q6h
Oxytetracycline	125, 250 mg cap, tab			
Oxytetracycline, calcium	125 mg/5 ml syrup	PO	40-50 mg/kg/day	q6h
Oxytetracycline HCl	125, 250 mg cap			
Oxytetracycline HCl Terramycin®	50, 100, 250 mg vials with 2% lidocaine	IM	15-25 mg/kg/day	q8-12h
Paromomycin sulfate Humatin®	250 mg cap 125 mg/5 ml syrup	PO	30 mg/kg/day	q8h
Penicillin G, benzathine Bicillin®	3 million unit 10 ml vial; 1, 1.5 and 2 ml syringes containing 600, 000 u/ml	IM	50,000 u/kg	1 dose
Penicillin G, potassium generic	125, 150, 250, 500 mg tab 125 250, 500 mg/5 ml syrup 1, 2, 10, 20 million unit vials	PO IM, IV	25-50 mg/kg/day 100,000-250,000 u/kg/day	q6-8h q4h

Generic and Trade® Names	Dosage Forms	Route	Dosage	Interval
Penicillin G, procaine Wycillin®	0.3, 0.6, 1.2. 2.4 million unit vial	IM	25,000-50,000 u/kg/day	q12-24h
Penicillin G, sodium	5 million unit vial	IM, IV	100,000-250,000 u/kg/day	q4h
Penicillin V Betapen-VK®, Pen-Vee K® Veetids®, generic	125, 250, 500 mg tab 125, 250 mg/5 ml sol'n 125, 250 mg/5 ml drops	PO	25-50 mg/kg/day	q6-8h
Pentamidine isethionate Pentam 300®, NebuPent®	300 mg vial	IV	4 mg/kg/day	q24h
Piperacillin Pipracil®	2, 3, 4 g vials	IV	200-300 mg/kg/day (Not approved for children)	q4-6h
Piperacillin/Tazobactam Zosyn®	3 g PIP/375 mg TAZ vial	IV	3 g PIP/375 mg TAZ (adult dosage)	q6h
Polymyxin B sulfate Aerosporin®	50 mg (500,000 unit) vial	IM, IV	3-4.5 mg/kg/day	q6h (IM); continuous infusion (IV)
Praziquantel Biltricide®	600 mg 3-scored tab	PO	50-75 mg/kg/day	q8h
Pyrantel pamoate Antiminth®	250 mg/5 ml susp	PO	11 mg/kg	1 dose
Pyrazinamide	500 mg tab	PO	30 mg/kg/day	q12-24h

78

Atabrine®

Drug	Preparation	Dosage	Route	Frequency
Ribavirin Virazole®	6 g vial	1 vial by SPAG-2 aerosol generator	Inhalation	q24h
Rifabutin Mycobutin®	150 mg cap	300 mg/day (adult dosage)	PO	q12-24h
Rifampin Rifadin®, Rimactane®	150, 300 mg cap 600 mg vial	10-20 mg/kg/day (max 600 mg)	PO IV	q12-24h
Rimantadine Flumadine®	100 mg tab 50 mg/5 ml syrup	5 mg/kg/day (max 150 mg/day)	PO	q24h
Spectinomycin HCl Trobicin®	2, 4 g vials	30-40 mg/kg	IM	1 dose
Streptomycin sulfate	1, 5 g vials	20-30 mg/kg/day	IM	q12h
Sulfadiazine	0.3, 0.5 g tab	120-150 mg/kg/day	PO	q4-6h
Sulfadiazine, sodium	2.5 g amp	100 mg/kg/day	SC, IV	q6-8h
Sulfadoxine and pyrimethamine Fansidar®	500 mg SDX + 25 mg PMA scored tab	(See Section IX)	PO	
Sulfamethizole Thiosulfil Forte®	0.5 g tab	30-45 mg/kg/day	PO	q6h
Sulfamethoxazole Gantanol®, generic	0.5 g tab 0.5 g/5 ml susp	50-60 mg/kg/day	PO	q12h
Sulfasalazine Azulfidine®, generic	500 mg tab	30-60 mg/kg/day	PO	q4-8h

Generic and Trade® Names	Dosage Form	Route	Dosage	Interval
Sulfisoxazole Gantrisin®, generic	0.5 g tab 0.5 g/5 ml susp or syrup	PO	120-150 mg/kg/day	q4-6h
Tetracycline Achromycin®, Sumycin®, generic	250, 500 mg cap, tab 125 mg/5 ml syrup 125, 250 mg/5 ml susp	PO	25-50 mg/kg/day	q6h
Thiabendazole Mintezol®	500 mg chewable, scored tab 500 mg/5 ml susp	PO	50 mg/kg/day	q12h
Ticarcillin disodium Ticar®	1, 3, 6 g vials	IV	200-300 mg/kg/day	q4-6h
Ticarcillin and clavulanate potassium Timentin®	3/0.1, 3/0.2 g vials	IV	200-300 mg/kg/day (not approved for children)	q4-6h
Tobramycin sulfate Nebcin®, generic	20, 80 mg, 1.2 g vials	IV, IM	3-6 mg/kg/day (cystic fibrosis 7-10)	q8h
Trifluridine Viroptic®	1% ophthal. sol'n	Topical	1 drop	q2h
Trimethoprim Proloprim®, Trimpex®, generic	100 mg scored tab	PO	4 mg/kg/day (not approved for children)	q12h
Trimethoprim-Sulfamethoxazole Bactrim®, Septra®, Sulfatrim® generic	80 mg TMP/400 mg SMX tab 160 mg TMP/800 mg SMX tab 40 mg TMP/200 mg SMX/5 ml susp	PO	8-12 mg TMP/ 40-60 mg SMX/kg/day; (20 mg TMP/100 mg SMX/kg/day for Pneumocystis)	q12h
	400 mg TMP/2000 mg SMX amp	IV		q6h

Drug	Preparation	Dosage	Frequency
Troleandomycin Tao®	250 mg cap	25-40 mg/kg/day	q6h
Vancomycin HCl Vancocin®, Vancoled®	1 g bottle 125, 250 mg cap	10-50 mg/kg/day	q6h
	500 mg vial	40 mg/kg/day (meningitis 60)	q6h
Vidarabine Vira-A®	3% ophthalmic ointment	Approx 1 cm of ointment	q3h
	1 g vial	10-30 mg/kg/day	q24h
Zalcitabine HIVID®	0.375, 0.750 mg tab	2.25 mg/day (adult dosage; given with zidovudine)	q8h
Zidovudine Retrovir®	100 mg cap 50 mg/5 ml syrup	See page 40	q6h

XI. ALPHABETICAL LISTING OF TRADE NAMES

[**Trade Name** (Drug Company)--Generic Name]

-A-

Achromycin (Lederle)
--Tetracycline

Aerosporin (Burroughs Wellcome)
--Polymyxin B

Amikin (Apothecon)
--Amikacin

Amoxil (SmithKline Beecham)
--Amoxicillin

Ancef (SmithKline Beecham)
--Cefazolin

Ancobon (Roche)
--Flucytosine

Antiminth (Pfizer)
--Pyrantel pamoate

Aralen (Winthrop)
--Cloroquine

Aralen with Primaquine (Winthrop)
--Cloroquine/primaquine

Atabrine (Winthrop)
--Quinacrine

A/T/S (Hoechst-Roussel)
--2% erythromycin sol'n (Topical)

Augmentin (SmithKline Beecham)
--Amoxicillin/clavulanate potassium

Aureomycin (Lederle)
--Chlortetracycline (Topical)

Azactam (Bristol-Myers Squibb)
--Aztreonam

Azo Gantanol (Roche)
--Sulfamethoxazole/phenazopyridine

Azo Gantrisin (Roche)
--Sulfisoxazole/phenazopyridine

Azulfidine (Pharmacia)
--Sulfasalazine

- B -

Bacitracin (Quad)
--Bacitracin

Bactocill (SmithKline Beecham)
--Oxacillin

Bactrim (Roche)
--Trimethoprim/sulfamethoxazole

Bactroban (SmithKline Beecham)
--Mupirocin (Topical)

Benemid (Merck)
--Probenecid

Betapen-VK (Apothecon)
--Penicillin V

Biaxin (Abbott)
--Clarithromycin

Bicillin (Wyeth-Ayerst)
--Benzathine penicillin G

Biltricide (Miles)
--Praziquantel

- C -

Ceclor (Lilly)
--Cefaclor

Cedax (Schering)
--Ceftibuten

Cefanix (Apothecon)
--Cephalexin

Cefadyl (Apothecon)
--Cephapirin

Cefizox (Fujisawa)
--Ceftizoxime

Cefobid (Roerig)
--Cefoperazone

Cefotan (Zeneca)
--Cefotetan

Ceftin (Allen & Hanburys)
--Cefuroxime axetil

Cefzil (BristolMyers Squibb)
--Cefprozil

Chibroxin (Merck)
--Norfloxacin ophthal. sol'n

Chloromycetin (Parke-Davis)
--Chloramphenicol

Cipro (Miles)
--Ciprofloxacin
Claforan (Hoechst-Roussel)
--Cefotaxime
Cleocin (Upjohn)
--Clindamycin
Cloxapen (SmithKline Beecham)
--Cloxacillin
Coly-Mycin (Parke-Davis)
--Colistin
Cytovene (Syntex)
--Ganciclovir

- D -
Dapsone USP (Jacobus)
--Dapsone
Daraprim (Burroughs Wellcome)
--Pyrimethamine
Declomycin (Lederle)
--Demeclocycline
Diflucan (Roerig)
--Fluconazole
Doryx (Parke-Davis)
--Doxycycline
Duricef (Mead Johnson)
--Cefadroxil
Dycill (SmithKline Beecham)
--Dicloxacillin
Dynapen (Apothecon)
--Dicloxacillin

- E -
E. E. S. (Abbott)
--Erythromycin ethylsuccinate
Elimite cream (Herbert)
--Permethrin 5% (Topical)
E-Mycin (Boots)
--Erythromycin
ERYC (Parke-Davis)
--Erythromycin
Erygel (Herbert)
--2% erythromycin gel (Topical)
EryPed (Abbott)
--Erythromycin ethylsuccinate
Ery-Tab (Abbott)
--Erythromycin

Erythrocin Lactobionate (Abbott)
--Erythromycin lactobionate
Erythrocin Stearate (Abbott)
--Erythromycin stearate
Erythromycin Base Filmtab (Abbott)
--Erythromycin
Erythromycin Stearate (Lederle)
--Erythromycin stearate
Eryzole (Alra)
--Erythromycin ethylsuccinate/
   sulfisoxazole acetyl

- F -
Fansidar (Roche)
--Sulfadoxine/pyrimethamine
Flagyl (Searle)
--Metronidazole
Floxin (Ortho)
--Ofloxacin
Flumadine (Forest)
--Rimantadine
Fortaz (Glaxo)
--Ceftazidime
Foscavir (Astra)
--Foscarnet
Fulvicin (Schering)
--Griseofulvin
Fungizone (Bristol-Myers Squibb)
--Amphotericin B
Furacin (Roberts)
--Nitrofurazone (Topical)
Furadantin (Roberts)
--Nitrofurantoin
Furoxone (Roberts)
--Furazolidone

- G -
Gantanol (Roche)
--Sulfamethoxazole
Gantrisin (Roche)
--Sulfisoxazole
Garamycin (Schering)
--Gentamicin
Geocillin (Roerig)
--Carbenicillin indanyl
Grifulvin V (Ortho)
--Griseofulvin

Grisactin (Wyeth-Ayerst)
--Griseofulvin
Gris-PEG (Herbert)
--Griseofulvin

- H -
Hiprex (Marion Merrell Dow)
--Methanamine hippurate
HIVID (Roche)
--Zalcitabine
Humatin (Parke-Davis)
--Paromomycin

- I -
Ilosone (Dista)
--Erythromycin estolate
Ilotycin (Dista)
--Erythromycin
Ilotycin Gluceptate (Dista)
--Erythromycin gluceptate
INH (Ciba)
--Isoniazid

- K -
Kantrex (Apothecon)
--Kanamycin
Keflex (Dista)
--Cephalexin
Keflin (Lilly)
--Cephalothin
Keftab (Dista)
--Cephalexin
Kefurox (Lilly)
--Cefuroxime
Kefzol (Lilly)
--Cefazolin

- L -
Lamprene (Geigy)
--Clofazimine
Laniazid (Lannett)
--Isoniazid
Lariam (Roche)
--Mefloquine
Lincocin (Upjohn)
--Lincomycin

Lorabid (Lilly)
--Loracarbef
Lotrimin (Schering)
--Clotrimazole (Topical)

- M -
Macrodantin (Proctor & Gamble)
--Nitrofurantoin
Mandelamine (Parke-Davis)
--Methenamine mandelate
Mandol (Lilly)
--Cefamandole
Maxaquin (Searle)
--Lomefloxacin
Mefoxin (Merck)
--Cefoxitin
Mepron (Burroughs Wellcome)
--Atovaquone
Metric-21 (Fielding)
--Metronidazole
Mezlin (Miles)
--Mezlocillin
Minocin (Lederle)
--Minocycline
Mintezol (Merck)
--Thiabendazole
Monistat (Ortho; Janssen)
--Miconazole
Monocid (SmithKline Beecham)
--Cefonicid
Myambutol (Lederle)
--Ethambutol
Mycelex (Miles)
--Clotrimazole
Mycitracin (Upjohn)
--Neomycin/bacitracin (Topical)
Mycobutin (Pharmacia)
--Rifabutin
Mycostatin (Apothecon)
--Nystatin

- N -
Nafcil (Apothecon)
--Nafcillin
Nebcin (Lilly)
--Tobramycin

84

NebuPent (Fujisawa)
--Pentamidine aerosol
NegGram (Winthrop)
--Nalidixic acid
Neosporin (Burroughs Wellcome)
--Neomycin, polymyxin B (Topical)
Netromycin (Schering)
--Netilmicin
Niclocide (Miles)
--Niclosamide
Nix Creme Rinse (Burroughs Wellcome)
--Permethrim 1% (Topical)
Nizoral (Janssen)
--Ketoconazole
Noroxin (Merck)
--Norfloxacin

- O -

Omnipen (Wyeth-Ayerst)
--Ampicillin
Ornidyl (Marion Merrell Dow)
--Eflornithine

- P -

Pathocil (Wyeth-Ayerst)
--Dicloxacillin
PCE Dispertab (Abbott)
--Erythromycin particles in tablets
Pediazole (Ross)
--Erythromycin ethylsuccinate/
  sulfisoxazole acetyl
Penetrex (Rhone-Poulenc Rorer)
--Enoxacin
Pentacef (SmithKline Beecham)
--Ceftazidime
Pentam 300 (Fujisawa)
--Pentamidine isethionate
Pen-Vee K (Wyeth-Ayerst)
--Penicillin V
Pipracil (Lederle)
--Piperacillin
Plaquenil (Winthrop)
--Hydroxychloroquine
Polycillin (Apothecon)
--Ampicillin

Polymox (Apothecon)
--Amoxicillin
Polysporin (Burroughs Wellcome)
--Polymyxin B/bacitracin (Topical)
Polytrim Ophthalmic Solution (Allergan)
--Trimethoprim and polymyxin B
  (Topical)
Primaxin (Merck)
--Imipenem-cilastatin
Principen (Apothecon)
--Ampicillin
Proloprim (Burroughs Wellcome)
--Trimethoprim
Prostaphlin (Apothecon)
--Oxacillin
Protostat (Ortho)
--Metronidazole
Pyrazinamide (Lederle)
--Pyrazinamide

- R -

Retrovir (Burroughs Wellcome)
--Zidovudine
Rifadin (Marion Merrell Dow)
--Rifampin
Rifamate (Marion Merrell Dow)
--Rifampin/isoniazid
Rimactane (Ciba)
--Rifampin
Rimactane/INH Dual Pack (Ciba)
--Rifampin/isoniazid
Rocephin (Roche)
--Ceftriaxone

- S -

Septra (Burroughs Wellcome)
--Trimethoprim/sulfamethoxazole
Seromycin (Lilly)
--Cycloserine
Sodium Sulamyd (Schering)
--Sodium sulfacetamide (Topical)
Spectrobid (Roerig)
--Bacampicillin
Sporanox (Janssen)
--Itraconazole

Staphcillin (Apothecon)
--Methicillin
Sulfatrim (Barre)
--Trimethoprim-sulfamethoxazole
Sumycin (Apothecon)
--Tetracycline
Suprax (Lederle)
--Cefixime
Symmetrel (DuPont/Merck)
--Amantadine

- T -

Tao (Roerig)
--Troleandomycin
Tazicef (SmithKline Beecham)
--Ceftazidime
Tazidime (Lilly)
--Ceftazidime
Tegopen (Apothecon)
--Cloxacillin
Terramycin (Roerig)
--Oxytetracycline
Thiosulfil Forte (Wyeth-Ayerst)
--Sulfamethizole
Ticar (SmithKline Beecham)
--Ticarcillin
Tice BCG Vaccine (Organon)
--BCG Vaccine
Timentin (SmithKline Beecham)
--Ticarcillin/clavulanate
Topicycline (Roberts)
--Tetracycline (Topical)
Trecator-SC (Wyeth-Ayerst)
--Ethionamide
Trimox (Apothecon)
--Amoxicillin
Trimpex (Roche)
--Trimethoprim
Trobicin (Upjohn)
--Spectinomycin

- U -

Ultracef (Bristol-Myers Squibb)
--Cefadroxil

Unasyn (Roerig)
--Ampicillin/sulbactam
Unipen (Wyeth-Ayerst)
--Nafcillin
Urex (3M)
--Methenamine hipprate
Urobiotic (Roerig)
--Oxytetracycline, sulfamethizole/
  phenazopyridine
Uroquid-Acid (Beach)
--Methenamine/sodium acid phosphate

- V -

Vancocin (Lilly)
--Vancomycin
Vancoled (Lederle)
--Vancomycin
Vantin (Upjohn)
--Cefpodoxime proxetil
Veetids (Apothecon)
--Penicillin V
Velosef (Apothecon)
--Cephradine
Vermox (Janssen)
--Mebendazole
Vibramycin (Roerig, Pfizer)
--Doxycycline
Vibra-Tabs (Pfizer)
--Doxycycline
Videx (Bristol-Myers Squibb)
--Didanosine
Vioform (Ciba)
--Iodochlorhydroxyquin (Topical)
Vira-A (Parke-Davis)
--Vidarabine
Virazole (ICN)
--Ribavirin
Viroptic (Burroughs Wellcome)
--Trifluridine (Ophthalmic)

- W -

Wyamycin S (Wyeth-Ayerst)
--Erythromycin stearate
Wycillin (Wyeth-Ayerst)
--Penicillin G procaine

Wymox (Wyeth-Ayerst)
--Amoxicillin

- Y -

Yodoxin (Glenwood)
--Iodoquinol (formerly
  diiodohydroxyquin)

- Z -

Zefazone (Upjohn)
--Cefmetazole
Zinacef (Glaxo)
--Cefuroxime
Zithromax (Pfizer)
--Azithromycin
Zolicef (Apothecon)
--Cefazolin
Zosyn (Lederle)
--Piperacillin/tazobactam
Zovirax (Burroughs Wellcome)
--Acyclovir

XII. ANTIBIOTIC THERAPY IN PATIENTS WITH RENAL FAILURE

Most antimicrobials are excreted primarily by the kidneys; therefore, when significant renal functional impairment is present, either downward adjustments in dosages must be made or the intervals between doses must be lengthened. Exceptions are drugs such as chloramphenicol that are metabolized to antibiotically inactive conjugates and those excreted primarily by the liver, such as nafcillin and ceftriaxone.

Degrees of dosage adjustment necessary for treating patients with renal failure are as follows: Major adjustments in dosage and dosing intervals are necessary for treating renal failure patients with aminoglycosides, flucytosine and vancomycin. No adjustments in dosage are necessary in the use of amphotericin B, cefoperazone, chloramphenicol, cloxacillin, dicloxacillin, doxycyline, erythromycin, isoniazid, metronidazole, minocycline, nafcillin and rifampin. For other antibiotics minor to moderate adjustments are necessary. For details, see **Pocket Manual of Drug Use in Clinical Medicine**, 4th ed, by D. Craig Brater, 1989. Publisher: B.C. Decker, Inc.

The most satisfactory way to use drugs in children with decreased renal function is by monitoring the antibiotic concentrations in serum. The customary initial loading dose is given. Initially, until antibiotic assay results are available, one makes estimates of appropriate dosage based on past experience of rates of excretion related to the degree of renal failure. Three or four serum specimens are collected at intervals over a 12-24 hour period for assay of antibiotic content. The serum half-life is estimated. The interval of dosing is every three half-lives for patients with moderate renal dysfunction and every two half-lives for those with severe renal failure; subsequent dosages are two-thirds or one-half, respectively, of the initial loading dose.

Patients undergoing dialysis need additional doses after the procedure if a substantial amount of drug is removed by dialysis. With peritoneal dialysis < 10% of drug is removed in the case of most antibiotics. The exceptions are aminoglycosides (20-25%), cefazolin and cefuroxime (20%), moxalactam and vancomycin (15-20%).

Removed by Hemodialysis	Beta-lactams	Other Drugs
> 50%	Many cephalosporins (see exceptions below), imipenem	Acyclovir, aminoglycosides, flucytosine, isoniazid, spectinomycin, sulfonamides, trimethoprim
20 - 50%	Most penicillins (see exceptions below), aztreonam cefaclor, ceforanide, cefapirin, moxalactam	Ethambutol, metronidazole, vancomycin
< 10%	Cefixime, cefonicid, cefoperazone, cefotetan, cloxacillin, dicloxacillin, methicillin, nafcillin, oxacillin	Amphotericin B, fluoroquinolones, macrolides, miconazole, polymyxins, tetracyclines

XIII. DILUTIONS OF ANTIBIOTICS FOR INTRAVENOUS USE

Notes:
1. Manufacturers' recommendations for dilution of antibiotics for intravenous use sometimes are not appropriate for pediatric patients because of volumes of fluid that are unsuitably large for the desired time of infusion. The dilutions given below should result in convenient volumes, and they are well-tolerated in terms of not causing irritation of veins.
2. The volumes of fluid in the tubing between the "piggyback" and the patient is approximately 15 ml. Therefore, in small babies who have slow rates of infusion, there may be a considerable delay before the antibiotic solution reaches the patients. It is recommended that either (a) the antibiotic solution be injected retrograde into the tubing via a three-way stopcock, or (b) that sufficient fluid be withdrawn from the tubing to allow antibiotic in the "piggyback" to enter the tubing.
3. Check the manufacturer's instructions for compatible IV solutions.

Antibiotics	Recommended Final Concentration for Administration	Usual Duration of Infusion
Penicillin G	Infants: 50,000 u/ml Large Child: 100,000 u/ml	10-20 min
Aztreonam	20 mg/ml	10-20 min
Other beta-lactam antibiotics	100 mg/ml	10-20 min
Chloramphenicol	125 mg/ml	10-20 min
Amikacin, clindamycin, kanamycin, lincomycin	6 mg/ml	15-30 min
Gentamicin, netilmicin, tobramycin	10 mg/ml	15-30 min
Vancomycin, imipenem	5 mg/ml	60 min
Metronidazole	5-8 mg/ml	60 min
Trimethoprim-sulfamethoxazole	0.64 TMP-3.2 SMX/ml (5 ml amp in 125 ml D5W)	60 min
Vidarabine	0.45 mg/ml	12-24 hr
Acyclovir, ganciclovir	7 mg/ml	1-3 hr
Amphotericin B	0.1 mg/ml	2-6 hr

XIV. MAXIMUM DOSAGES FOR LARGE CHILDREN

Infants and young children have a large volume of distribution of many antibiotics in the body. This means that, in order to achieve good serum concentrations, we give larger doses based on body weight or surface area than are given to adults. The following dosages of commonly used drugs should not be exceeded except in special circumstances. (See p. 7 for oral therapy of serious infections.)

Maximum Daily Dosage	Antimicrobials
ORAL FORMULATIONS	
4-8 g	Sulfisoxazole
2-3 g	Amoxicillin, ampicillin, carbenicillin, cephalexin, cephradine, chloramphenicol, cloxacillin, cyclacillin, lincomycin, nafcillin, oxacillin, penicillin G or V, tetracycline
1-2 g	Cefaclor, cefprozil, cefuroxime axetil, ciprofloxacin, clindamycin, dicloxacillin, erythromycin, metronidazole
0.5-1.2 g	Loracarbef, trimethoprim
400 mg	Cefixime, cefpodoxime
PARENTERAL FORMULATIONS	
30-40 g	Carbenicillin
18-24 g	Azlocillin, mezlocillin, piperacillin, ticarcillin
10-12 g	Ampicillin, cefotaxime, ceftizoxime, cephalothin, methicillin, moxalactam, nafcillin, oxacillin
6-8 g	Aztreonam, ceftazidime
4-6 g	Cefamandole, cefoperazone, cefazolin, cefuroxime
2-4 g	Ceftriaxone, chloramphenicol, clindamycin, erythromycin, metronidazole, spectinomycin, vancomycin
1-2 g	Amikacin, cefonicid, ceforanide, streptomycin, tetracycline
0.75-1 g	Kanamycin, lincomycin
300 mg	Gentamicin, netilmicin, tobramycin
20 million units	Penicillin G
4.8 million units	Penicillin G, procaine
2.4 million units	Penicillin G, benzathine

XV. DOSAGES BASED ON BODY SURFACE AREA

Antibiotic dosages calculated on the basis of body weight are not always appropriate for obese and malnourished patients. (Obese patients would have excessively high serum concentrations, and malnourished patients would have lower than desired serum concentrations.) For such patients dosages calculated from body surface area are preferred.

Calculation of body surface area (**J Pediatr** 93:62, 1978)

B.S.A. (m^2) = wt $(kg)^{0.5378}$ x ht $(cm)^{0.3964}$ x 0.024265, which can be solved using logarithms on a pocket calculator as:

log B.S.A. = log wt x 0.5378 + log ht x 0.3964 + log 0.024265

Antibiotics (IM or IV)	Each Dose/m^2	Interval	Amt/m^2/24 hrs
Aminoglycoside			
Amikacin, kanamycin	200 mg	q8h	600 mg
gentamicin, netilmicin,			
tobramycin	60 mg	q8h	180 mg
Beta-Lactams			
Penicillin G (meningitis)	1,750,000 u	q4h	10,500,000 u
Penicillin G (others)	450,000 u	q4h	2,700,000 u
Ampicillin, methicillin,			
oxacillin, cephalothin	1.4 g	q6h	5.6 g
Ceftriaxone	1.4 g	q12h	2.8 g
Ceftazidime, moxalactam	1.4 g	q8h	4.2 g
Nafcillin, cefamandole,			
cefotaxime, ceftizoxime	1.05 g	q6h	4.2 g
Cefazolin, cefuroxime	0.8 g	q8h	2.4 g
Cefonicid, ceforanide	0.55 g	q12h	1.1 g
Carbenicillin	4 g	q6h	16 g
Ticarcillin, azlocillin,			
mezlocillin, piperacillin	2.5 g	q6h	10 g
Aztreonam	0.8 g	q6h	3.2 g
Imipenem	0.55 g	q6h	2.2 g
Miscellaneous			
Chloramphenicol (meningitis)	0.7 g	q6h	2.8 g
Chloramphenicol (others)	0.45 g	q6h	1.8 g
Metronidazole	280 mg	q8h	840 mg
(Sulfamethoxazole	0.5 g	q8h	1.5 g)
(Trimethoprim	100 mg	q8h	300 mg)
Vancomycin (CNS infection)	0.425 g	q6h	1.7 g
Vancomycin (others)	0.275 g	q6h	1.1 g
Zidovudine	160 mg	q6h	640 mg

XVI. ADVERSE REACTIONS TO ANTIMICROBIAL AGENTS

It is a good rule of clinical practice to be suspicious of an adverse drug reaction when a patient's clinical course deviates from the expected. This section focuses on reactions that require close observation or laboratory monitoring either because of their frequency or because of their severity. For detailed listings of reactions, consult the package inserts.

Beta-Lactam Antibiotics. The most feared reaction to penicillins, anaphylactic shock, is extremely rare and there is no absolutely reliable means of predicting its occurrence. The commercially available skin testing material, benzylpenicilloylpolylysine (Pre-Pen®), should be used in conjunction with the Minor Determinant Mixture (MDM) and penicilloic acid skin testing, but the latter two are not yet commercially available. A dilute solution of penicillin G (10,000 u/ml) can be used as a skin test material in place of MDM. If the scratch test and intradermal test with 0.01 ml are negative, penicillin of the same lot number should be used for administration to the patient. (Be prepared to treat anaphylaxis.) If there is question about the allergic status one can use a desensitization schedule (See Section III). The monobactam, aztreonam, does not exhibit cross-sensitization with penicillins and cephalosporins.

Ampicillin and other aminopenicillins cause minor adverse effects frequently. Oral or diaper area candidiasis, diarrhea and morbilliform, blotchy "ampicillin rashes" are common. The latter is not allergic in origin and is not a contraindication to subsequent use of ampicillin or of any other penicillin. Diarrhea is somewhat less common with amoxicillin, bacampicillin and cyclacillin and more common with Augmentin®. Rarely beta-lactams cause serious, life-threatening pseudomembranous enterocolitis due to suppression of normal bowel flora and overgrowth with *Clostridium difficile*. Drug fever is probably more common with ampicillin than with other penicillins. Serum sickness is uncommon. Pancytopenia is rare and reversible neutropenia and thrombocytopenia occasionally occur with any of the beta-lactams.

Nephrotoxicity is probably most common with methicillin (approximately 5%) but has been reported with all the penicillins (rarest with nafcillin). Laboratory monitoring should be performed. Hemorrhagic cystitis occurs mainly in poorly hydrated patients receiving large dosages and is probably a direct irritant effect of the large concentrations of drug in urine. It disappears even with continued use of the antibiotic when the patient's urine output increases. Carbenicillin and ticarcillin interfere with platelet function but generally do not cause clinical bleeding problems. Hypokalemia is more common with these drugs than with other beta-lactams. Mezlocillin and piperacillin appear to have similar adverse effects to carbenicillin and ticarcillin with the exception that mezlocillin has the least effect on platelet function.

Imipenem-cilastatin has similar adverse effects to other beta-lactams. In addition, patients occasionally have CNS reactions (convulsions, hallucinations, altered affect). Convulsions are most likely in the elderly or in patients with CNS disease.

The cephalosporins for oral use are generally better tolerated than the penicillins. The cephalosporins can cause a direct Coombs' reaction in the blood, but this is of no known clinical significance. Most cephalosporins are painful on IM injection and can cause phlebothrombosis with IV administration. Cefazolin and cefuroxime are better tolerated IM, and cefamandole and cephradine appear to cause fewer problems on IV use than the others. Cefaclor has been associated with a transient serum sickness-like reaction (rash, arthralgia); the cause is unknown. Similarly, a serum sickness-like reaction has been reported with IV use of cephapirin. Cefoperazone and cefamandole can cause a disulfiram (Antabuse)-like effect; patients should avoid alcohol, including elixirs. Prolonged prothrombin time and bleeding episodes have also been attributed to those drugs. It is treatable (and probably preventable) with vitamin K. The third generation cephalosporins cause profound alteration of normal flora on mucosal surfaces, and all have caused pseudomembranous colitis on rare occasions. Ceftriaxone commonly causes loose stools, but it is rarely severe enough to require stopping therapy. Ceftriaxone can cause sludging in the gallbladder which, on rare occasions, causes symptoms and jaundice; this is reversible after stopping the drug. Ceftriaxone is also reported to displace bilirubin from albumin-binding sites.

Aminoglycosides. Any of the aminoglycosidic aminocyclitol antibiotics can cause serious nephrotoxicity and ototoxicity. (The closely related aminocyclitol, spectinomycin, is safer in this respect.) The newer aminoglycosides (amikacin, tobramycin, gentamicin and netilmicin) are generally safer than kanamycin, streptomycin or neomycin. In animal studies, netilmicin is the least ototoxic. Monitor all patients receiving aminoglycoside therapy for renal toxicity with periodic urinalyses and determinations of the BUN and creatinine and be alert to ototoxicity. It is common practice to measure the serum concentration one-half to one hour after a dose to make sure one is in a safe and therapeutic range and a trough serum concentration immediately preceding a dose. Monitoring is especially important in patients with any degree of renal insufficiency. Elevated trough concentrations (>2 μg/ml for gentamicin, netilmicin and tobramycin and >10 μg/ml for amikacin and kanamycin) should be avoided. Aminoglycosides potentiate botulinum toxin.

The "loop" diuretics (ethacrynic acid, furosemide, piretanide and bumetanide) potentiate the ototoxicity of the aminoglycosides. The "non-loop" diuretics (hydrodiuril, mercuhydrin and mannitol) do not interact with aminoglycosides to produce ototoxicity.

The aminoglycosides are well tolerated via intramuscular and intravenous routes of administration. Minor side effects such as rashes, drug fever, etc. are rare.

Chloramphenicol. The most feared toxicity of chloramphenicol, irreversible aplastic anemia, is very rare. It has been said that aplastic anemia is more likely with oral than with parenteral chloramphenicol, but it is hard to document that claim and it is probably incorrect. Regardless of the route of administration, laboratory monitoring for hematologic toxicity should be carried out in all patients treated with chloramphenicol. Transient pharmacologic bone marrow depression occurs in almost all patients receiving large dosages (> 75 mg/kg/day) of chloramphenicol. As long as the absolute neutrophil count remains more than 1,500 per μl and the platelet count above 100,000 per μl one can continue to administer chloramphenicol if it is necessary. These hematologic changes reverse rapidly when the drug is stopped.

The "gray syndrome" with fatal circulatory collapse is due to excessive accumulation of chloramphenicol in neonates secondary to delayed conjugation (because of inadequate glucuronyl transferase activity) and poor renal excretion of unconjugated chloramphenicol. Chloramphenicol should not be used in neonates unless there are no suitable alternative drugs; dosage must be restricted and, ideally, one would monitor serum concentrations (therapeutic range 10-25 μg/ml). Phenobarbitol induces glucuronidative enzymes so that patients receiving phenobarbitol may require larger than normal doses of chloramphenicol. Rifampin has a similar effect. Concomitant phenytoin administration often causes accumulation of chloramphenicol in serum, which may reach a toxic concentration; conversely, accumulation of phenytoin to toxic concentrations has also been reported. Other drugs metabolized by the liver, such as theophylline, acetaminophen and isoniazid, could have similar effects.

Minor side effects such as nausea and diarrhea are rare. With prolonged use (principally in children with cystic fibrosis), optic neuritis and peripheral neuritis have occurred. Alteration of normal respiratory and gastrointestinal flora may lead to infection with opportunistic bacteria or fungi. Drug fever is rare.

Tetracyclines. Tetracyclines should be used infrequently in pediatric patients because the legitimate applications are uncommon diseases (rickettsial infections, brucellosis), with the exception of acne, chlamydial infections and Lyme disease in teenagers. Side effects include minor gastrointestinal disturbances, photosensitization, angioedema, browning of the tongue, glossitis, pruritis ani, and exfoliative dermatitis. The diarrhea associated with tetracycline administration may be a direct irritant effect or due to alteration of normal GI flora with overgrowth of opportunistic bacteria or fungi. Alterations in normal respiratory tract flora produced by tetracycline increase the risk of superinfections by staphylococci and other opportunistic organisms.

Toxic effects from tetracyclines involve virtually every organ system. Hepatic and pancreatic injury have occurred with accidental overdosage and in patients with renal failure. (Pregnant women are particularly at risk for hepatic injury.) Tetracyclines are deposited in growing bones and teeth with depression of linear bone growth and dental staining and defects in enamelization in deciduous and permanent teeth. This effect is dose-related and the risk extends up to 8 years of age. Patients taking outdated, degraded tetracycline can develop a Fanconi renal syndrome. Pseudotumor cerebri of unknown cause has rarely been seen in young infants who receive normal therapeutic doses. Minocycline causes dose-related vestibular toxicity in adults. Tetracycline is painful and irritative when injected into muscle and thrombophlebitis occurs if the drug is given IV too rapidly.

Macrolides. Erythromycin is one of the safest antimicrobial agents. It commonly produces nausea and epigastric distress at dosages greater than 40 mg/kg/day. Decreased hearing which returns to normal after discontinuation of the drug has been reported several times. Alteration of normal flora is generally not a problem, but oral or perianal candidiasis occasionally develops. Transient cholestatic hepatitis is a rare complication that occurs with approximately equal frequency among the various formulations of erythromycin, but the estolate is said to pose a particular risk to pregnant women. Intramuscular administration of erythromycin is painful and irritative. IV doses should be administered slowly (1-2 hr).

Clindamycin and lincomycin can cause nausea, vomiting and diarrhea. Pseudomembranous colitis due to suppression of normal flora and overgrowth of *Clostridium difficile* is uncommon, especially in children, but potentially serious. Urticaria, glossitis, pruritis and skin rashes occur occasionally. Serum sickness, anaphylaxis and photosensitivity are rare as are hematologic and hepatic abnormalities.

The newer macrolides, azithromycin and clarithromycin, are less likely than erythromycin to cause gastrointestinal side effects.

Polymyxins. Polymyxin B and polymyxin E (colistin sulfate and colistimethate) are mainly of historic interest and are rarely used now except in topical preparations. With parenteral administration the major toxicity is to the kidneys. They also cause various neurological reactions such as flushing, dizziness, ataxia, diplopia, dysphagia, and paresthesias. Neuromuscular blockade with respiratory arrest has occurred. Hematologic or hepatic toxicity has rarely been attributed to the polymyxins. Oral colistin sulfate is well tolerated with few side effects.

Antituberculous Drugs. Gastrointestinal irritation is very common with aminosalicylic acid. Hypersensitivity reactions such as drug fever, skin rashes and arthralgias are relatively common. Hepatic and renal toxicity is rare as are various hematologic abnormalities. Prolonged treatment with aminosalicylic acid can produce goiter. Isoniazid is generally well tolerated and hypersensitivity reactions are rare. Peripheral neuritis (preventable or reversed by pyridoxine administration) and mental aberrations from euphoria to psychosis occur more often in adults than in children. Mild elevations of ALT in the first weeks of therapy, which disappear with continued administration, are common. Rarely, frank hepatitis develops. Rifampin also can cause hepatitis; it is more common in patients with pre-existing liver disease or in those taking large dosages. Risk of hepatic damage increases when rifampin and isoniazid are taken together in dosages more than 15 mg/kg of each daily. Gastrointestinal, hematologic and neurologic side effects of various types have been observed on occasion. Hypersensitivity reactions are rare. Pyrazinamide can cause hepatic damage which appears to be dose-related.

Antifungal Drugs. Amphotericin B, flucytosine, miconazole and ketoconazole can produce serious adverse reactions. Amphotericin B is probably the most toxic antimicrobial drug in clinical use. Chills, fever, flushing and headaches are the commonest of the many adverse reactions. Some degree of decreased renal function occurs in up to 80% of patients given amphotericin B. Anemia is common and, rarely, hepatic toxicity and neutropenia occur.

The major toxicity of flucytosine is bone marrow depression and this seems to occur mainly in patients with a pre-existing hematologic disorder and in those treated with irradiation or cancer chemotherapeutic drugs. Mild gastrointestinal upset, mental confusion and vertigo sometimes occur. Renal function should be monitored.

There is little experience with the parenteral preparation of miconazole in children but it appears to be only slightly less toxic than amphotericin B. Patients receiving miconazole should be monitored for hematologic, hepatic and renal toxicity.

Ketoconazole has produced hepatic damage on rare occasions. The most common side effect is gastric distress; this can often be alleviated by dividing the daily dose. Gynecomastia is not rare in adult males.

Fluconazole is generally well tolerated. Gastrointestinal symptoms, rash and headache occur occasionally. Transient, asymptomatic elevations of hepatic enzymes have been reported.

Vancomycin. Vancomycin can cause phlebitis if the drug is injected rapidly or in concentrated form. Vancomycin is said to have the potential for ototoxicity and nephrotoxicity, but it is difficult to document these effects in children. It was reported that vancomycin potentiated the nephrotoxicity of aminoglycosides but further study showed that this was incorrect. Hepatic toxicity is rare. Neutropenia has been reported. If the drug is infused too rapidly (fewer than 60 minutes) a transient rash of the upper body with itching may occur from histamine release ("red man syndrome"). It is not a contraindication to continued use and is less likely if the infusion rate is at least 60-120 minutes. Vancomycin in conjunction with anesthesia has been reported to cause hypotension and hypothermia.

Sulfonamides and Trimethoprim. The commonest adverse reaction to sulfonamides is a hypersensitivity rash. Rarely, Stevens-Johnson syndrome occurs; it was most common with very long-acting sulfas that are no longer marketed. The frequency and types of reactions to the trimethoprim-sulfamethoxazole combination are said to be the same as with sulfamethoxazole alone, but it is not clear whether Stevens-Johnson syndrome is caused more often by the combination than by sulfamethoxazole alone. Neutropenia and anemia occur occasionally. The rash caused by TMP/SMX appears to be more common in patients taking large dosages. Rash is common in adults with AIDS. Mild depression of platelet counts occurs in approximately one-half the patients treated with sulfas or trimethoprim-sulfamethoxazole but this rarely produces clinical bleeding problems. Sulfa drugs can precipitate hemolysis in patients with glucose-6-phosphate dehydrogenase deficiency. Crystalline aggregates of sulfa drugs may be deposited in the kidneys or ureters and cause acute nephropathy (most likely with sulfadiazine and least likely with trisulfapyrimidines). Adequate urine output and alkalinization of the urine minimize the risk. Drug fever and serum sickness are infrequent hypersensitivity reactions. Hepatitis with focal or diffuse necrosis is rare.

Fluoroquinolones. All quinolone and fluoroquinolone drugs cause cartilage damage in toxicity studies in various immature animals, although there are no conclusive data indicating similar toxicity in young children. Studies are underway to evaluate this, but until those results are available there has been reluctance to use the fluoroquinolones in pediatric patients. Reported side effects include gastrointestinal symptoms, dizziness, headaches, tremors, confusion, seizures and rash. Hepatic toxicity is rare. Large dosages may precipitate hypoglycemia in the elderly. Severe hemolytic anemia occurred with temofloxacin with a frequency of approximately 1:10,000 patients; because of this the drug was withdrawn from the market.

XVII. ADVERSE INTERACTIONS OF DRUGS

Antibiotic	Interacting Drug	Adverse Effect
Acyclovir	Probenecid	Poss incr acyclovir toxicity
Amantadine	Anticholinergics	Hallucinations, nightmares, confusion
Amikacin (See Aminoglycosides)		
Aminoglycosides	Amphotericin B	Incr nephrotoxicity
	Anti-*Pseudomonas* penicillins (if renal failure)	Decr aminoglycoside serum conc
	Cephalosporins	Poss incr nephrotoxicity
	Digoxin	Poss decr digoxin effect
	Ethacrynic acid, furosemide, bumetanide	Incr ototoxicity
	Methotrexate	Poss incr methotrexate toxicity
	Neuromuscular blocking agents; magnesium sulfate	Incr neuromuscular blockage
Amphotericin B	Aminoglycosides	Incr nephrotoxicity
	Curariform drugs	Incr curariform effect
	Digitalis drugs	Incr digitalis toxicity
	Miconazole	Decr anti-*Candida* effect
	Neuromuscular blocking agents	Hypokalemia
Ampicillin	Oral contraceptives	Decr contraceptive effect
	Allopurinol	Incr incidence of rash
Cephalosporins	Alcohol (cefamandole, cefoperazone, moxalactam)	Antabuse-like effect
	Aminoglycosides	Poss incr nephrotoxicity
	Ethacrynic acid, furosemide	Incr nephrotoxicity
	Aspirin, heparin (moxalactam)	Poss incr bleeding risk

Antibiotic	Interacting Drug	Adverse Effect
	Anticoagulants (moxalactam)	Incr anticoagulant effect
Chloramphenicol	Acetaminophen	Incr chloramphenicol toxicity
	Barbiturates	Incr barbiturate effect; Decr chloramphenicol effect
	Dicumarol	Incr anticoagulant effect
	Phenytoin	Altered pharmacology of both drugs
	Rifampin	Decr chloramphenicol effect
Ciprofloxacin	Theophylline, cyclosporine	Incr theophylline, cyclosporine
	Antacids	Decr ciprofloxacin absorption
Clindamycin, Lincomycin	Neuromuscular blocking agents	Incr neuromuscular blockade
	Diphenoxylate-atropine	Incr diarrhea, colitis
Cycloserine (See Isoniazid)		
Erythromycin	Anticoagulants	Incr anticoagulant effect
	Digoxin	Incr digoxin effect
	Theophylline	Incr theophylline effect
	Carbamazepine	Incr carbamazepine effect
	Seldane	Cardiotoxic
Furazolidone	Alcohol	Antabuse-like effect
	Alpha-adrenergic amines	Incr hypertensive effect
Gentamicin (See Aminoglycosides)		

Antibiotic	Interacting Drug	Adverse Effect
Griseofulvin	Oral anticoagulants	Decr anticoagulant effect
	Phenobarbital	Decr griseofulvin effect
Isoniazid	Aluminum antacids	Decr isoniazid effect
	Anticoagulants	Poss incr anticoagulant effect
	Carbamazepine	Incr toxicity of both drugs
	Cycloserine	Dizziness, drowsiness
	Phenytoin	Incr phenytoin toxicity
	Rifampin	Incr hepatotoxicity
Kanamycin (See Aminoglycosides)		
Ketoconazole	Antacids	Decr ketoconazole effect
	Cimetidine	Decr ketoconazole effect
	Cyclosporine	Incr cyclosporine effect
	Erythromycin	Cardiotoxic
Lincomycin (See Clindamycin)		
Metronidazole	Alcohol	Antabuse-like reaction
	Anticoagulants	Incr anticoagulant effect
	Phenobarbital	Decr metronidazole effect
Miconazole (See Amphotericin B)		
Nalidixic acid	Oral anticoagulants	Incr anticoagulant effect
Netilmicin (See Aminoglycosides)		
Quinacrine	Alcohol	Antabuse-like effect

Antibiotic	Interacting Drug	Adverse Effect
Rifampin	Anticoagulants, barbiturates, beta-adrenergic blockers, contraceptives, corticosteroids, diazepam, digitoxin, hypoglycemics, quinidine	Decreased effect of interacting drug
	Chloramphenicol	Decr chloramphenicol effect
	Isoniazid	Incr hepatotoxicity
	Methadone	Methadone withdrawal symptoms
Spectinomycin	Lithium	Incr lithium toxicity
Streptomycin (See Aminoglycosides)		
Sulfonamides	Oral anticoagulants	Incr anticoagulant effect
	Hypoglycemics	Incr hypoglycemia
	Methotrexate	Poss incr methotrexate toxicity
	Phenytoin	Incr phenytoin effect
	Thiopental	Incr thiopental effect
Tetracyclines	Antacids, bismuth subsalicylate, iron, zinc sulfate	Decr tetracycline effect
	Phenytoin, barbiturates and carbamazepine	Decr doxcline effect
	Oral contraceptives	Decr contraceptive effect
	Lithium	Incr lithium toxicity
Thiabendazole	Theophylline	Incr theophylline effect
Tobramycin (See Aminoglycosides)		
Trimethoprim-sulfamethoxazole	Anticoagulants	Incr anticoagulant effect
	Cyclosporine	Incr nephrotoxicity
Troleandomycin	Carbamazepine	Incr carbamazepine effect
	Oral contraceptives	Jaundice
	Theophylline	Incr theophylline effect
Vidarabine	Allopurinol	Incr vidarabine toxicity

XVIII. INDEX OF DISEASES

Note: Only diseases are indexed. For alphabetical listings of microorganisms, antibiotics and trade names see Sections VII, X and XI, respectively.

103

NOTES

NOTES

Mac Oair⁵⁴ 5948